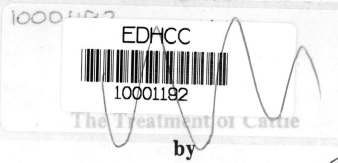
The Treatment of Cattle

by

Homoeopathy

Other works by George Macleod

THE TREATMENT OF HORSES BY HOMOEOPATHY
A VETERINARY MATERIA MEDICA
CATS: HOMOEOPATHIC REMEDIES
DOGS: HOMOEOPATHIC REMEDIES
GOATS: HOMOEOPATHIC REMEDIES

The Treatment of Cattle
by
Homoeopathy

by
G. Macleod
M.R.C.V.S., D.V.S.M.

VETERINARY MEMBER OF THE FACULTY OF HOMOEOPATHY

VETERINARY CONSULTANT TO MESSRS. A. NELSON & CO.
HOMOEOPATHIC PHARMACY, LONDON

VETERINARY CONSULTANT TO THE
BRITISH HOMOEOPATHIC ASSOCIATION

VETERINARY CONSULTANT TO THE
HOMOEOPATHIC DEVELOPMENT FOUNDATION

Index by
Maurice Prior

THE C. W. DANIEL COMPANY LTD.
1 CHURCH PATH, SAFFRON WALDEN
ESSEX, ENGLAND

First published in Great Britain by
The C. W. Daniel Company Ltd.
1 Church Path, Saffron Walden
Essex, England

©G. MACLEOD 1981
Reprinted 1991

ISBN 0 85207 247 3

Set in 10/12 point Times
by White Crescent Press Ltd., Luton, Beds

Produced by
Ennisfield Print & Design
Wapping, London

Contents

Introduction

In compiling this outline of common cattle diseases, those which are subject to control under the Diseases of Animals Acts and Orders have been deliberately omitted for obvious reasons. Also certain other specific diseases have been left out simply because any treatment, conventional or homoeopathic is uneconomical and animals suffering from them are better culled, e.g. Johnes Disease and certain others which while not enzootic in Britain, may be subject to control in other countries.

A section on Materia Medica has been included relating to remedies mentioned in the text which I hope will enable the reader new to homoeopathy to grasp a little of the essentials of each remedy, its origins and range of action, etc. These are the summaries only, with references to the conditions discussed. For a fuller description of remedies the reader should consult a standard Materia Medica.

Finally, I would like to thank Mr John Ainsworth of Ainsworth's Homoeopathic Pharmacy and his staff and also Miss Nora Macleod for giving me much of their time to typing the manuscript and for persevering in the face of some rather unusual nomenclature.

Lindfield
August 1979

Preface

This outline of the homoeopathic approach to the commoner diseases of cattle has been written as a guide for all those who have asked for some information on this alternative system of medicine as it applies to the cow and her calf. It will readily be appreciated that many conditions which might call for treatment in the smaller animals have been omitted, e.g. serious injuries, and others which are not economic to treat.

When a veterinary surgeon practices the use of homoeopathic medicine and is asked why he does so, he may give one of several answers. A generation ago the simple answer was that results were good, but as the years passed, and the changing pattern of disease became evident, an emphatic answer was that homoeopathic treatment has no unpleasant or dangerous side-effects, while still achieving successful results. The difference between the conventional approach and the homoeopathic leads to the rejection by homoeopaths of the idea that destruction of bacteria is the main aim of the physician, because it is not the illness as such one has to treat, but the patient's reaction to it.

How then can the homoeopathic system be employed to the benefit of the livestock farmer? There are two approaches to this question and to animal health in general, viz. (1) Preventive medicine and (2) the therapeutic approach, or the emergency treatment of individual cases. It is generally accepted that a programme of preventive medicine is the ideal state of affairs and homoeopathy is well suited to this approach, possessing a wide range of nosodes, or oral vaccines, for use against most conditions, including those for the control of which there are no conventional vaccines available.

Nosodes and Oral Vaccines.
For the reader who is new to homoeopathy, it will be necessary to define the terms 'nosode' and 'oral vaccine', and explain fully the difference between them and conventional vaccines, which are administered by injection.

A nosode is a disease product obtained from any affected part of the system in a case of illness, frequently from lymph nodes or from respiratory secretions, e.g. nasal discharges in a case of catarrhal fever, and thereafter potentised. In specific, i.e. bacterial, viral or protozoal disease the causative organism may or may not be present and the efficacy of the nosode in no way depends on the organism being present. The response of the tissues to invasion by bacteria or other antigens results in the formation of substances which are in effect the basis of the nosode.

An oral vaccine is prepared from the actual organism which is associated with the disease in question, and may derive from filtrates containing only the exotoxins of the bacteria, or from emulsions containing both bacteria and their toxins. These filtrates and emulsions are then potentised and become oral vaccines. Nowadays it is the custom to use the terms 'nosodes' and 'oral vaccines' synonymously

Auto-nosodes.
This particular type of nosode is prepared from material provided by the patient alone, e.g. pus from a chronic sinus or fistula, and after potentisation used for the treatment of the same patient. Many examples of this could be given, but I think it is sufficient to explain the theory. Auto-nosodes are usually employed in refractory cases where well-indicated remedies have failed to produce the desired response, and frequently they give striking results.

Bowel Nosodes.
In the section on calf diseases, reference is made to these nosodes in connection with the diseases coli-bacillosis and coccidiosis. They represent a special group of potentised oral vaccines derived from certain bowel flora – the non-lactose fermenting bacteria. They have a complementary effect on certain homoeopathic remedies, and may be used in conjunction with them in the treatment of disease. Sycotic Co. which is mentioned in the text is one of a group of five or six which have various claims. The others need not concern us here.

Nosodes can also be used therapeutically either on their own or with indicated remedies. In acute conditions, e.g. in calf scour, it may be necessary to give the nosode three times a day for two days, or even more frequently during the course of 24 hours. For more chronic conditions and in cases of convalescence after infectious disease, a single dose may suffice.

Many farmers today are concerned not only with the increasing cost of conventional drugs but also with their side-effects in many cases, and with the build-up of resistant strains of bacteria due to the continued, and often indiscriminate use of antibiotics. This is particularly true of the attempted control of mastitis by the repeated application of intra-mammary agents containing one or other of the indicated drugs. While, therefore, this book, which outlines the homoeopathic approach to disease in cattle will appeal to the already converted, it is hoped that the unprejudiced newcomer will be sufficiently encouraged after reading it to investigate this system of medicine for himself, and partake of its undoubted benefits. The aim of the homoeopathic approach is to build up the health of the herd and increase the resistance of its individual members to disease, and, in consequence to increase the milk output; as the healthier the cow is, the more milk it will produce, and the quality of milk will also improve. The first six months are the most important in any animal's life. What happens then will determine for good or ill much of its later life. Calves which are subjected to a programme of preventive medicine based on the use of nosodes against the commoner diseases will eventually grow into heifers and steers, and achieve weight gain at an earlier age than they otherwise would. This is especially important from the point of view of the beef farmer.

Administration of Remedies.

Homoeopathic remedies for use in cattle are usually marketed in one gram vials incorporating the remedy in a sugar-granule base. The remedy (in tincture form) is simply added to the granules and allowed to soak in, after which it is stable and remains active for many months and sometimes years if stored under the proper conditions. These vials are referred to as 'veterinary doses'. When treating an animal, the contents of the vial should be emptied directly on to the animal's tongue, and allowed to dissolve in the saliva. It is not necessary for the animal to swallow the granules, as homoeopathic remedies possess the advantage over conventional drugs in being absorbed through the palate or tongue. Some farmers and stockmen find this procedure tedious, but a little practice will soon make the attendant proficient, and the results are worth the little trouble involved. It is not proposed that this procedure should be followed on a herd basis. For large numbers of animals it may be necessary to add the remedy to the drinking water and for this purpose remedies can be obtained in tincture form using a 5ml dose (see section on Mastitis) This method is particularly suitable for dealing with large numbers of dairy cows in a programme of preventive medicine.

For those owners who prefer it, remedies may also be administered by injection provided certain safeguards or precautions are observed. Remedies are sold as single or compound sealed vials, each being a single dose, but it is essential to point out that if this method of administration is followed, a new sterile syringe must be used for each vial and strict asepsis observed. They are much more expensive than the veterinary doses referred to above if bought in the United Kingdom, but more economical in Germany, where they are frequently used and accordingly cheaper to manufacture.

Potencies of Remedies.

The potencies of the various remedies outlined in the text are offered as a general guide, and it may be found necessary according to the condition, not only to vary them or use a different strength, but also to extend the period of time over which they are given for longer than is suggested in the text.

Also, very acute conditions may require higher strengths of remedies than are generally outlined. I make it a general rule that the more acute the condition, the higher the potency needed, while chronic states involving tissue change are catered for by the lower potencies. This is not a hard and fast rule, as other practitioners of homoeopathic medicine have different veiws. This may appear confusing to the newcomer, but the more he becomes familiar with the subject the easier it will be for him to arrive at the optimum potency for each remedy and condition.

The Nature of Homoeopathic Remedies.

Homoeopathic remedies are derived from all natural sources, animal or biological, mineral or plant, and their preparation is an expert subject best left to a qualified pharmacist. Some ill-informed people believe that remedies are simple dilutions, but this is not the case. The attenuation, or small dose of the remedy, is dependent on the technique known as potentisation. Any substance can become a homoeopathic remedy, but it is of use only after the pharmacist has refined the crude product in order to develop its inherent properties, and render its medicinal energy avialable for use. Preparation of the remedy includes first dilution, and then succussion. The latter is essential to the procedure, and consists of a vigorous shaking by special equipment. Those dilutions prepared in this way are referred to as potencies, and are used in either of two ways: (1) the decimal system used largely in Germany, and expressed by the numerals/ letters x and D, and (2), the centesimal system favoured more in Britain and the U.S.A., and expressed by the letter c. They differ only in the degree of dilution and succussion carried out at each stage. The more we dilute and succuss the remedy, the more the energy is released, so that the curative properties of the drug are retained, while all poisonous or unpleasant side-effects of the crude drug are lost, e.g., the active principles of poisonous plants such as Aconitum Napellus or Atropa Belladonna are rendered innocuous after the third centesimal potency. The power of the attenuated dose lies in its ability to permeate the cell membrane, and accepted laboratory techniques have produced proof of the activity of infinitesimal doses of homoeopathic remedies in potency. Without elaborating this further, we need only note that this use of the minute, or infinitesimal dose, is an essential corollary to the homoeopathic principle of 'let likes be cured by likes'.

Owners who are themselves homoeopaths will be aquainted with the 'sameness' of the remedies as regards their appearance and taste, but to others, to whom homoeopathy is new, I would draw attention to the following simple rules. The medicines all look the same and taste the same. It is important to realise that they are all different, and that one remedy cannot be substituted for another. Do not therefore remove any vials from their boxes until they are required for use. As remedies are purchased with their name and potency labelled on the box, it is a good practice to write these again on the bottom of the box to prevent mistakes arising. The remedies should be kept in their boxes when not in use, and stored in a cool, dry atmosphere away from sunlight and strong-smelling substances such as camphor, creosote or carbolic. Do not, therefore, store the remedies in farm outhouses.

1. Diseases of the Respiratory System

1. Epistaxis – Nose-bleed. This condition when due to injury is less common than in the horse.

ETIOLOGY. Haemorrhage due to trauma can be associated with bull-holders and other mechanical devices. Bleeding may be caused by abscesses or tumours and also occurs in certain septicaemic conditions, and in poisoning by bracken and clover.

SYMPTOMS. The bleeding may be confined to one nostril only when it is usually associated with local lesions; or it may be bilateral when generalised upset is present. The character of the blood may indicate venous or arterial haemorrhage and care must be taken to differentiate local bleeding from that arising from pulmonary involvement.

TREATMENT.
1. *Arnica 6c.* When haemorrhages arise as a result of local injury, arnica should always be employed. Dose: in acute cases one dose should be given every hour for four doses. When the injury is of longer duration, two doses of a higher potency, e.g. 1m, are indicated, each dose being 24 hours apart.
2. *Belladonna 200c.* If there is involvement of the central nervous system this remedy should be considered, symptoms such as full pulse and dilated pupils determining its use. Dose: one dose ever hour for four doses.
3. *Ammonium Carbonicum 30c.* Beef animals in good condition may respond well to this remedy, rather than thinner animals of the dairy type. Dose: one dose three times daily for two days.

2. Coryza or Catarrhal Rhinitis. This condition is an inflammation of the nasal passages and is invariably associated with infection of one kind or another.

ETIOLOGY. A Primary cause may be exposure to cold or damp weather as happens when cattle are left out at night in late autumn. Young animals may show symptoms when they are confined in cold damp pens. Specific Rhinitis is associated with infectious disease.

SYMPTOMS. There may be an initial rise of temperature which, in calves, may reach 105°F. Nasal mucous discharge accompanies lachrymation due to conjunctival inflammation. The discharge soon becomes muco-purulent and coughing takes place. The mucosa of the nasal passages becomes red and swollen. Swelling of the sub-maxillary lymph glands is frequently seen.

TREATMENT. The treatment outlined here relates only to simple uncomplicated Rhinitis. Coryza associated with specific disease and secondary to pneumonia or bronchitis will be dealt with under these conditions.

1. *Aconite 30c.* This is a useful preliminary remedy and should be given early in the febrile stage if possible. Dose: one dose every half-hour for six doses.

2. *Arsenicum Album 1m.* Indicated when there is an accompanying conjunctivitis and signs of respiratory involvement. The nasal discharge may be acrid. Dose: one dose every hour for four doses.

3. *Silicea 200c.* Thickening of the nasal mucosa, associated with hypertrophy calls for this remedy. Dose: one dose daily for one week.

4. *Pulsatilla 30c.* When the inside of the nose becomes encrusted with scales, this remedy may help. There may be purulent lachrymation. Dose: one dose three times daily for three days.

5. *Mercurius Corrosivus 30c.* Disease of the nasal bones calls for mercury. The discharge contains blood and mucus and shows a greenish tinge. Dose: one dose daily for five days.

6. *Allium Cepa 6c.* Bland discharges early in the affection indicate the need for this remedy. Lachrymation is common and the eyes appear red. Dose: one dose every half-hour for four doses.

7. *Hydrastis 30c.* When the discharge becomes catarrhal and yellow. Dose: one three times daily for two days.

8. *Dulcamara 200c.* This remedy should be considered when the condition arises as a result of exposure to a fall in temperature

after a warm day, as frequently happens in late summer or early autumn. Dose: one every three hours for four doses.

3. Chronic Rhinitis – Chronic Nasal Catarrh. This condition may be associated with a chronic pneumonia or pharyngitis and can accompany abscess formation due to specific organisms.

SYMPTOMS. Respiration becomes difficult due to a chronic thickening of the nasal mucosa. This is accompanied by a purulent nasal discharge which may be thick at times. Throat glands may become swollen leading to further embarrassment of respiration.

TREATMENT.
1. *Kali Bichromicum 30c.* Purulent yellow discharge of a tough, stringy nature calls for this remedy. Dose: one three times daily for three days.
2. *Hydrastis 6c.* Thick catarrhal discharges are associated with this remedy. Discharge is free-flowing. Dose: one twice daily for four days.
3. *Mercurius Solubilis 30c.* Discharges are greenish and may be tinged with blood. Caries of nasal bones may be present. Dose: one dose twice daily for five days.
4. *Silicea 200c.* When this remedy is indicated the purulent discharge is thin and greyish looking. The nasal bones may be thickened. Dose: one daily for seven days.

4. Sinusitis. Acute inflammation of the sinuses is relatively uncommon in cattle, but a chronic form frequently follows dehorning.

SYMPTOMS. Shortly after dehorning under unsuitable conditions a suppurative inflammation may set in and progresses to a longer-lasting purulent sinusitis. Proliferation of the sinus lining may accompany a necrosis of the bone in severe cases. There may be head shaking and a rise in temperature in the initial stage. Purulent discharge from the nose is seen early on but later this may be absent.

TREATMENT.
1. *Hepar Sulphuris 6x.* Employed in this low potency the remedy will hasten elimination of purulent material. The pus is usually thin and free-flowing. Dose: one three times daily for four days.

2. *Silicea 200c.* Proliferation of sinus lining may call for this remedy. The accompanying discharge is thin, greyish and foul-smelling. Dose: one per day for one week.
3. *Kali Bichromicum 30c.* Retention and inspissation of purulent material is associated with this remedy. The pus appears as yellow, stringy masses. Dose: one three times daily for four days.
4. *Mercurius Corrosivus 200c.* Indicated when suspected caries of bone has taken place, the overlying facial bones being puffy and soft. Pus discharged is greenish and may be tinged with blood. Dose: one daily for seven days.
5. *Hydrastis 30c.* When the discharge is more catarrhal and mucoid with less purulent involvement. Dose: one three times daily for five days.

5.   Laryngitis. Inflammation of the laryngeal area is frequently associated with other respiratory conditions such as bronchitis and pneumonia. It may be acute or chronic.

ETIOLOGY.   Acute laryngitis often accompanies colds and exposure to inclement weather.

SYMPTOMS.   There is lack of appetite and sometimes a fall in milk yield in severe cases. A dry painful cough accompanies the condition which may extend down the respiratory tract. The chronic form is often secondary to more serious disease such as actinobacillosis or pulmonary abscess. It leads to narrowing of the laryngeal opening and produces difficulty in inspiration.

TREATMENT.
1. *Aconite 30c.* Will be helpful in the acute form if given early. Dose: one every hour for four doses.
2. *Spongia Tosta 6c.* A useful remedy for controlling laryngeal cough. Dose: one three times daily for three days.
3. *Mercurius Cyanatus 30c.* If there is an accompanying membrane of the throat, this is the remedy of choice. Dose: one three times daily for two days.
4. *Sanguinaria 6c.* A good remedy for controlling laryngeal oedema. Dose: one three times daily for three days.
5. *Drosera 9c.* Spasmodic coughing accompanying the condition

may call for this remedy. Dose: one three times daily for four days.

6. *Rhus Toxicodendron 1m.* This is a useful remedy when the throat is dark red and there is accompanying lachrymation. Dose: one twice daily for four days.

6. Tracheitis. Inflammation of the windpipe may be either acute or chronic.

ETIOLOGY. Predisposing factors include damp or unhygienic buildings leading to the establishment of infection, pasteurella organisms and viruses being commonly implicated.

SYMPTOMS. Fever may rise to 105° or 106°F. Respirations become increased and there is a frequent dry cough which later may become moist. The cough is easily induced by pressure on the trachea. The acute form may lead into a chronic state which in turn can produce more serious disease such as bronchitis or pneumonia. A mucous cough is the main symptom of the chronic form and if the disease process spreads down to the lung tissue signs of pneumonia become evident.

TREATMENT.
1. *Bryonia 30c.* Useful for controlling the dry cough of the acute stage. Dose: one three times daily for two days.
2. *Aconite 6x.* For the initial feverish stage. Dose: one every half-hour for four doses.
3. *Dulcamara 30c.* When arising as a result of exposure to damp conditions, especially in autumn or late summer. Dose one three times daily for three days.
4. *Drosera 9c.* A useful remedy for controlling spasmodic cough. Dose: one three times daily for three days.

7. Congestion of Lungs. This condition may arise from an increased blood-supply when it is termed active, or when there is interference with blood supply-passive congestion.

ETIOLOGY. Exposure to cold weather is a common cause, as also is transportation over long distances. It may accompany diseased conditions such as hepatitis or severe mastitis.

SYMPTOMS. There may be a rapid rise in temperature, breathing becomes laboured and frothy saliva is evident, accompanied by a grunting sound when breathing out. The severity of the laboured breathing depends on the amount of fluid present.

TREATMENT.
1. *Aconite 6x.* For the early feverish stage. Dose: one every half-hour for four doses.
2. *Ammonium Causticum 30c.* Controls moist coughing. Dose: one three times daily for three days.
3. *Antimonium Tartaricum 30c.* For pneumonic complications accompanied by mucous râles. Dose: one three times daily for four doses.
4. *Apis Mel. 6c.* Helps control oedema. Dose: one every two hours for four doses.
5. *Antimonium Arsenicum 30c.* A valuable remedy when the congestion is worse on the left side. The patient frequently prefers to lie down and there may be an accompanying oedema of the brisket. Dose: one three times daily for one week.
6. *Ammonium Carbonicum 30c.* More suitable for right-sided congestion, usually venous in origin. Dose: one three times daily for one week.

8. Oedema of Lungs. This comes about when serum from blood-vessels finds its way into lung tissue.

ETIOLOGY. Any stress factor may produce this condition and can arise from anaphylactic reaction resulting from injection of foreign material, e.g. vaccines or sera.

SYMPTOMS. Sudden onset is accompanied by severe dyspnoea with frothy saliva abundant. The head is held low and thin mucus may run from the mouth. Grunting is common and auscultation reveals the presence of lung fluid in excess.

TREATMENT.
3. *Aesculus 30c.* A useful remedy when oedema arises as a result of passive congestion. Dose: one three times daily for three days.
2. *Ammonium Causticum 30c.* When there is an accompanying exhaustion or muscular weakness. Mucus is greatly increased. Dose: one three times daily for four days.

3. *Antimonium Tartaricum 6c.* When there is threatened pneumonia and mucus in abundance. Dose: one three times daily for three days.
4. *Apis Mel 30c.* Helps reduce the amount of fluid present. Dose: one hourly for four doses.
5. *Antimonium Arsenicum 30c.* For symptoms which appear to be worse on the left side. Dose: one every three hours for four doses.
6. *Ammonium Carbonicum 200c.* More suitable for oedematous involvement of the right chest. Dose: one twice daily for five days.

9. Haemorrhage from the Lungs. This is usually secondary to some serious condition.

ETIOLOGY. Any lung condition which leads to erosion of blood-vessels may produce lung haemmorhage, e.g. abscess formation due to Corynebacteria. The presence of lung tumour is also a factor.

SYMPTOMS. The blood may be bright red and frothy accompanied by difficult breathing. The condition is often due to a chronic underlying broncho-pneumonia and is often preceded by a history of nose bleeding.

TREATMENT.
1. *Aconite 30c.* Should be given if the condition arises suddenly accompanied by symptoms of stress. Dose: one every half-hour for four doses.
2. *Arnica 30c.* Frequently associated with heart complications. Dyspnoea severe. Dose: one three times daily for two days.
3. *Ipecacuanha 6c.* When there is an accompanying lack of appetite and nose-bleed. The slightest exertion produces expectoration of bright blood. Dose: one dose four times in 24 hours, for one day.
4. *Melilotus 6x.* Muscular weakness present. Frequently associated with clover poisoning. Dose: one every hour for four doses
5. *Millefolium 6c.* Palpitation with bright red blood. Sometimes associated with a chronic lung condition. Dose: one every three hours for four doses.
6. *Phosphorus 200c.* Repeated bouts of coughing and bleeding.

Blood rust-coloured and usually dependent on an underlying pneumonia. Dose: one dose night and morning for one week.

7. *Ficus Religiosa 6c.*   Another valuable remedy with symptoms of coughing and the production of bright red blood. Accompanying pulse rate is very weak. Dose: one three times daily for four days.

10.   Pneumonia. This may take various forms, e.g. broncho-pneumonia or acute virus or pasteurella pneumonia when the disease is more lobar in type. The lung lesion may arise suddenly or be insidious in onset.

ETIOLOGY.   Exposure to cold and damp are predisposing conditions. Fatigue and transportation are contributory factors. Infectious agents include viruses and sometimes pasteurella organisms and also corynebacteria.

SYMPTOMS.   A rise in temperature accompanies coughing, depression and lack of appetite. Respirations are greatly increased. Clear mucus appears on the nostrils, but this soon gives way to a more purulent discharge. Grunting and mouth breathing are present in severe cases. Percussion over the chest reveals dullness over the lower area, while emphysema is present over the upper area. Auscultation reveals a variety of sounds according to the degree of involvement.

TREATMENT.

1. *Aconitum 6x.*   Should be given early if possible. Dose: one every half-hour for four doses.
2. *Antimonium Tartaricum 200c.*   For moist coughing with patchy distribution of lung lesions. Frothy saliva. Dose: one three times daily for three days.
3. *Beryllium 30c.*   When symptoms are more severe than the clinical findings would suggest. Slight movement brings on coughing. Dose: one night and morning for four days.
4. *Bryonia 30c.*   When the animal is disinclined to move. Harsh sounds are heard over the pleura. The animal prefers to lie down. Dose: one three times daily for three days.
5. *Drosera 9c.*   Spasmodic cough is present. Has given particularly good results in young calves. Dose: one three times daily for three days.

6. *Lycopodium 200c.* When the condition is suspected of being secondary to digestive or hepatic disturbance. Breathing is very laboured involving independent movement of the nostrils. Dose: one every two hours for four doses.
7. *Phosphorus 1m.* When there is extensive consolidation of lung tissue together with rust-coloured sputum. Dose: one evey hour for four doses.
8. *Tuberculinum Aviare 200c.* Young animals may respond well to this remedy. The upper portions of the lungs are more frequently involved. Dose: one night and morning for three days.

11. Pulmonary Abscess. Suppurative Pneumonia. This may be part of a chronic pneumonia complicated by the presence of purulent foci.

ETIOLOGY. It may arise as a metastatic condition. Fatal pneumonias frequently end this way. Mastitis, metritis or some other severe septic state may give rise to metastases with resulting suppurative foci.

SYMPTOMS. Persistent cough and loss of condition supervene. There is usually lung bleeding and a purulent nasal discharge, the latter being common in calves as a sequel to enzootic pneumonia.

TREATMENT. Purulent Pneumonia is extremely difficult to treat effectively, but the following remedies may be of use.
1. *Hepar Sulph 200c or 1m.* A useful general remedy for septic states. Dose: one three times daily for five days.
2. *Carbo Vegetabilis 6c.* Neglected Pneumonia with purulent expectoration: useful in cases of threatened collapse. Dose: one three times daily for two days.
3. *Silicea 200c.* Poorly nourished animals showing greyish purulent expectoration may improve on this remedy. Dose: one dose daily for seven days.

12. Pleurisy. Inflammation of the pleura is seldom seen as a primary condition.

ETIOLOGY. Acute pleurisy is usually secondary to pneumonia or pericarditis, while a chronic form may be associated with lung conditions such as abscess or fusiformis infection of the liver.

SYMPTOMS. The acute form is of sudden onset accompanied by lack of appetite, rise in temperature and evidence of pneumonia over the chest wall. A rasping sound is heard on auscultation. Respirations are increased when secondary to pneumonia. Chronic pleurisy is most often secondary to traumatic pericarditis.

TREATMENT.
1. *Apis 6c.* Suitable for cases involving oedema of the pleural cavities. There may be an accompanying brisket oedema. Dose: one three times daily for three days.
2. *Arsenicum Iodatum 30c.* Chronic pleurisy may be relieved by this remedy. It is useful for cases which are slow to respond. Dose: one twice daily for seven days.
3. *Bryonia 6c.* The animal resents movement and prefers to lie down. Pressure over the chest relieves the pain. Dose: one every three hours for four doses.
4. *Kali Carbonicum 200c.* Pain is worse on the right side. There is early morning cough. Dose: one twice daily for five days.

13. Pulmonary Emphysema. This is seen as a sequel to pneumonia, extensive interstitial changes taking place in the lung tissue. It also arises as a result of continual respiratory distress such as severe dyspnoea.

CLINICAL SIGNS. Dyspnoea is a constant sign and may be of such intensity for the animal to exhibit mouth breathing. There is generally frothy saliva present and coarse râles are heard on auscultation. Sometimes emphysema is seen in the subcutaneous tissue. Rapid grunting breathing is usual along with sunken eyes and increased pulse rate in severe cases.

TREATMENT. This is not an easy condition to treat, but the following remedies may relieve the symptoms.
1. *Ammonium Carbonicum 6c.* Asthmatic coughing is made worse in warm conditions. Blood may be coughed up occasionally. Râles are worse on the right side. Dose: one three times daily for five days.
2. *Antimonium Arsenicum 6c.* Excessive dyspnoea with sounds worse on the upper left chest. The animal prefers to remain standing. Dose: one dose three times daily for one week.

3. *Arsenicum Album 1m.* For restless animals which show a desire to drink small quantities of water frequently. Symptoms such as coughing and dyspnoea become progressively more severe as night approaches. Dose: one per day for two weeks.
4. *Drosera 9c.* For milder cases showing spasmodic coughing and upper laryngeal distress. Dose: one three times daily for one week.
5. *Bryonia 30c.* The animal resents movement preferring to lie down and remain perfectly still. Pressure over the chest wall produces an amelioration of the symptoms. Dose: one twice daily for two weeks.
6. *Lobelia Inflata 30c.* Animal seems better on movement; worse after food. Frequent attacks of short coughing. Dose: one three times daily for one week.

14. Fog Fever. This is a form of pulmonary emphysema affecting both beef and dairy cattle.

ETIOLOGY. Seasonal factors play an important role in the development of the disease and allergic factors are considered to be the exciting cause.

CLINICAL FINDINGS. There are two forms of this condition, acute and chronic. In the acute type, symptoms appear shortly after susceptible animals are turned out on lush grazing in early autumn, when the predisposing factors operate in the presence of early morning mist. Severe difficulty in breathing is soon evident and foam-flecked, frothy saliva appears which can be copious at times. An anxious expression accompanies an increased heart rate. The tongue protrudes in severe cases. There is an expiratory grunt. Chronic forms are sometimes seen in winter, this type being associated with deep coughing and broncho-pneumonia.

TREATMENT.
1. *Antimonium Tartaricum 200c.* Indicated when there is moist coughing and abundant frothy saliva. Dose: one every two hours for four doses, followed by one daily for three doses.
2. *Apis Mellifica 6c.* This remedy will help control the pulmonary oedema. Dose: one every three hours for four doses.

3. *Bryonia 30c.*   If the animal resents movement and there is relief on percussion. Dose: one three times daily for three days.
4. *Drosera 9c.*   Useful in chronic forms where there is deep and protracted coughing. Dose: one three times daily for four days.
5. *Lycopodium 1m.*   When laboured respirations accompany digestive symptoms such as slight rumenal tympany. Pneumonia is sometimes severe. Dose: one every two hours for four doses.
6. *Phosphorus 200c.*   Indicated in the chronic form when pneumonia develops quickly. Respirations are short and rapid. Dose: one every two hours for four doses.

2. Diseases of the Circulatory System

A. The Heart.

1. Myocarditis. Inflammation of Heart Muscle.

ETIOLOGY. Myocarditis may arise as a result of toxic substances reaching the heart muscle during the course of severe infections.

SYMPTOMS. The heart rate is increased, while temperature may be raised slightly. Dilation of heart muscle may lead to weakening of the muscle wall with palpitation and variation in heart sounds.

TREATMENT.
1. *Digitalis 3x.* A useful remedy where there is dilation and variation in beat. Dose; one three times daily for two weeks.
2. *Crataegus 3x.* Should be given as a routine after toxic states to prevent damage to the muscle. Regulates heart beat. Dose: one three times daily for two weeks.
3. *Strophanthus 3x.* Weakness of heart muscle generally. Will aid diuresis in oedematous states. Is less cumulative than the other heart remedies and can therefore be given for longer periods. Dose: one twice daily for one month.

2. Endocarditis. Inflammation of the endothelial lining of the heart. May also involve the heart valves.

ETIOLOGY. Bacteria are usually implicated in Endocarditis and produce fibrinous deposits on the valves and thickening of the endothelium.

SYMPTOMS. There is usually a generalised infection present. Valvular involvement may lead to narrowing of the openings due to fibrinous growths. There is a distinct heart murmur present.

TREATMENT.
1. *Cactus Crandiflorus 6x.* Useful in incompetence of mitral valve. Very rapid heart action. Dose: one three times daily for one week.
2. *Convallaria 1x.* The least exertion brings on distress. Irregular rapid pulse. Dose: one three times daily for two weeks.
3. *Naja Tripudians 6c.* Associated with coldness of body, weak pulse and low tension. Especially useful after infectious disease. Dose: one three times daily for one week.

3. Pericarditis. Inflammation of the heart sac is usually accompanied by the effusion of serum into the sac. This fluid may change from sero-fibrinous to sero-purulent.

ETIOLOGY. It may be secondary to infection, or can be an extension from the pleura, accompanying chest injuries.

SYMPTOMS. On auscultation a friction sound is heard which is related to the heart's action. This may lessen as the heart sac fills with fluid. Accumulation of fluid leads to embarrassment of heart action and an increase in venous pressure which is evident in the appearance of a jugular pulse.

TREATMENT.
1. *Apis Mellifica 6c.* This remedy is helpful in controlling the effusion and amount of fluid into the heart sac. Dose: one three times daily for four days.
2. *Bryonia 30c.* If the condition is thought to have arisen as an extension of pleurisy. The animal resents movement preferring to lie down on the left side. Pressure over the heart area relieves symptoms. Dose: one three times daily for five days.
3. *Calcarea Fluorica 30c.* A useful remedy for relieving the stress on the heart muscle as a result of thickening of the heart sac. Dose: one daily for one week.

B. Phlebitis.
Inflammation of a vein may follow intravenous injection, or arise as a sequel to a blow or some other form of trauma.

SYMPTOMS. Acute phlebitis is attended by swelling and heat, followed by the formation of a thrombus or clot. This may occlude the vein in severe cases and is sometimes seen in the jugular vein when it then stands out as a thickened cord-like structure.

TREATMENT.
1. *Haemamelis 6c.*   A good general venous remedy. The eye and throat veins may be engorged. Dose: one twice daily for seven days.
2. *Lachesis 30c.*   Useful in acute stages. The skin surrounding the superficial veins may appear bluish or purple. Dose: one twice daily for five days.
3. *Vipera 12c.*   For acute cases showing constitutional symptoms such as involvement of liver with jaundice. Pressure on the affected veins causes resentment. Dose: one three times daily for five days.

3. Diseases of the Digestive System

1. Catarrhal or Simple Stomatitis. Inflammation of the mucous membrane of the mouth includes also involvement of gums and tongue.

ETIOLOGY. This condition may arise as a result of chemical or plant poisoning, or as an accompaniment to certain constitutional upsets, e.g. derangement of digestion.

SYMPTOMS. Salivation occurs and in severe cases this may be frothy. The mucous membrane of the mouth becomes red and swollen.

TREATMENT.
1. *Kali Chloricum 6c.* If there is an accompanying digestive upset; e.g. gastro-intestinal catarrh, this is a good remedy. Dose: one three times daily for four days.
2. *Mercurius Solubulis 30c.* If ropy salivation is the main symptom, this remedy may help. There is a tendency for the saliva to be blood-stained. Dose: one three times daily for two days.
3. *Nux Vomica 12x.* Suitable for cases which arise as a result of rumenal impaction. Dose: one four times daily for two days.
4. *Rhus Toxicodendron 1m.* A useful remedy for redness of the mucosa extending to the throat and associated with small vesicles. Dose: one twice daily for five days.

2. Phlegmonous Stomatitis. This is a more deep-seated inflammation, characterised by purulent discharge in many instances.

ETIOLOGY. May arise as a result of injury from burns or from infection in diseases such as mucosal disease and malignant catarrhal fever.

SYMPTOMS. There is evidence of pain when the animal attempts to eat. The tongue becomes severely swollen and profuse salivation occurs. The mucous membrane of the tongue and gums assumes a shiny appearance and may be bright red or bluish-red. Oedema of the sub-maxillary region may occur.

TREATMENT.
1. *Belladonna 1m.*   Useful when the mucosa is red and shiny. The skin is usually hot. Dose: one every three hours for four doses.
2. *Mercurius Corrosivus 200c.*   Purulent discharge, ropy saliva and membranous deposits call for this remedy. Dose: one three times daily for three days.
3. *Mercurius Cyanatus 6c.*   If the phlegmonous deposits extend to the throat leading to the formation of a greyish membrane. Dose: one three times daily for three days.
4. *Nitricum Acidum 200c.*   For ulceration accompanied by abundant froth and reddish-pink gums and papillae. There may be an accompanying ulceration of the nose. Dose: one three times daily for three days.

3.   Allergic Stomatitis.   This form is associated with the ingestion of certain harmful plants and is invariably accompanied by photo-sensitisation of unpigmented areas of skin and sometimes by jaundice. It frequently has a seasonal incidence, the majority of cases appearing in spring and autumn.

ETIOLOGY.   Both red and white clover have been implicated, while in some countries Lucerne or Alfalfa is blamed.

SYMPTOMS.   Small ulcerated lesions appear around the nostrils which become reddened. In severe cases, salivation is profuse accompanying erosion of the buccal mucous membrane which later show yellowish deposits. Conjunctivitis may occur. The skin lesions appear as bare patches which become moist and red and later crusty and leathery. Jaundice is frequently present.

TREATMENT.   The remedies mentioned already for stomatitis in general will be applicable here also. In addition the following remedies will aid the complicating conditions.
1. *Chelidonium 1m.*   Indicated when the skin and membranes of the eye appear dirty yellow. There may be an accompanying stiffness of the fore-quarters, especially the right. Dose: one night and morning for five days.

2. *Hypericum 1m.* Will aid the skin lesions to heal quickly. Pain in the lesions will be reduced helping to eliminate or reduce itching with consequent scratching. Dose: one dose per day for five days.
3. *Borax 6c.* When ulceration takes place on the dental pad and dorsum of the tongue. The animal is disinclined to move in a forward or downward manner. Dose: one dose twice daily for one week.

4. Inflammation of Salivary Glands. The glands involved are the parotid, sub-maxillary and sub-lingual.

ETIOLOGY. Abscess formation may lead to swelling of the parotid and sub-maxillary glands. Specific diseases such as actinobacillosis may involve these glands also, while phlegmonous stomatitis is involved in swelling of the sub-maxillary space extending to the gland.

SYMPTOMS. When the parotid gland is involved the region surrounding the gland becomes firm and the swelling extends to include the entire throat area. Heat is present in acute cases. The swelling interferes with swallowing and respiration: oedema of the sub-maxillary space occurs.

TREATMENT.
1. *Baryta Carbonicam 30c.* For young animals. Throat involvement is common. Dose: one twice daily for four days.
2. *Belladonna 1m.* The glands are hot, firm and hard. Pupils usually dilated with a hot skin and full pulse. Dose: one every hour for four doses.
3. *Hepar Sulphuris 30x.* Indicated when there is abscess formation. The gland is extremely sensitive to touch. Dose: one three times daily for two days.
4. *Phytolacca 6c.* For firm hard glands without abscess formation. Other neighbouring glands may be indurated. Dose: one three times daily for three days.
5. *Pulsatilla 30c.* Suitable more for right-sided parotitis. The tongue is usually dry. Dose: one twice daily for four days.

5. Acute Indigestion. This is usually a disturbance of physiological function, no pathological changes taking place.

ETIOLOGY.   Overeating is a frequent cause and this may relate to normal feed or to the animal having access to palatable foods such as grain or cake and eating too much of either. Damaged feeds may cause the condition. Early fermenting silage or new mown hay may produce symptoms if sufficient quantity is taken. Unthrifty animals or those suffering from certain mineral deficiencies may eat indigestible material with resulting stomach trouble. Young calves frequently suffer from indigestion from being fed poor hay or corn silage before their systems are adjusted to cope with such food.

SYMPTOMS.   Acute indigestion may be accompanied by tympany. Simple indigestion shows as lack of appetite with a slight increase in the rate of respiration. The faeces may be hard or watery depending on the nature of the food partaken. Rumenal contractions may be reduced when the dung is dry or increased when diarrhoea is present. Rumenal impaction produces a doughy feeling with reduced stomach movement. Severe overloading of the rumen may lead to toxaemia if treatment is not started early, symptoms of recumbency, sluggish reflexes and sub-normal temperature being usual.

TREATMENT.
1. *Abies Canadensis 6c.*   A useful remedy when overeating is the cause. Abdominal flatulence is common. Dose: one dose four times in 24 hours.
2. *Carbo Vegetabilis 6c.*   For toxaemic states, comatose symptoms being present. Dose: one every hour for four doses.
3. *Colchicum 6c.*   Rumenal tympany calls for this remedy. The origin frequently lies in too much green food. Dose: one every two hours for four doses.
4. *Nux Vomica 12x.*   Indicated when arising from indigestible fodder. Constipation is invariably present. Dose: one dose every two hours for three doses.

6.   Enteritis.   Acute inflammation of the intestinal tract.

ETIOLOGY.   It may follow acute indigestion or be secondary to some septic state such as mastitis or metritis.

SYMPTOMS.   Diarrhoea occurs with evidence of pain. The animal refuses food. Shreds of mucus may be present along with blood accompanied by straining.

TREATMENT.
1. *Aconite 30c.* Should be given early if possible. Will help combat shock and calm the patient. Dose: one every half-hour for four doses.
2. *Arsenicum Album 1m.* Restlessness and a worsening of the condition towards midnight calls for this remedy. The stool has a cadaverous odour. Dose: one every hour for four doses.
3. *Colocynthis 6c.* Symptoms of abdominal pain are prominent. The animal lies down and rises frequently. Blood may be present in the stool. Dose: one every half-hour for four doses.
4. *Croton Tiglium 30c.* Stools are watery and forcibly expelled. Dose: one dose every hour for five doses.
5. *Mercurius Corrosivus 200c.* Mucous, dysenteric stools having a slimy consistency. Symptoms are worse during night. Dose: one three times daily for three days.

7. Peritonitis. Inflammation of the peritoneum is rarely primary.

ETIOLOGY. It is usually a sequel to some condition such as gastritis, metritis or mastitis. Abscess of the liver may lead to it. Any septicaemic condition may also produce peritonitis.

SYMPTOMS. Lack of appetite accompanies a rise in temperature and pulse rate together with an increase in respirations. The back becomes arched and a painful grunt is present on expiration. The peritoneal covering can be felt as a hard board-like structure on deep pressure ove the sub-lumbar fossa.

TREATMENT.
1. *Aconite 6x.* Will relieve pain and anxiety if given early. Dose: one every hour for four doses.
2. *Belladonna 1m.* The animal has a high temperature, feels hot and has a staring look. Head shaking may occur. Dose: one every half-hour for five doses.
3. *Bryonia Alba 30c.* Tenderness over the abdomen is extreme. Sensitivity to touch. Very hard feeling on pressure. Dose: one four times in 24 hours.
4. *Cantharis 30c.* Severe inflammatory involvement of whole peritoneal covering. Blood in stools. Usually dependent on a basic cystitis or nephritis. Dose: one every half-hour for six doses.

5. *Rhus Tox 1m.* Relief is evident on movement. Redness of visible mucous membranes. Dose: one every two hours for five doses.

8. Bloat. Acute tympany of the rumen is a specific form of indigestion which can arise suddenly when gas in the rumen is produced faster than it is eliminated.

ETIOLOGY. Lush pastures in spring or autumn may result in outbreaks of bloat in the herd while large amounts of grain are also implicated. A reduced intake of roughage will contribute to bloat as the rumen depends on a sufficient quantity for its proper function.

SYMPTOMS. A fullness or swelling, small at first, appears over the left sub-lumbar fossa. This swelling increases rapidly as the rumen fills with gas. The animal becomes increasingly distressed and anxious-looking. Soon the swelling becomes hard and tense, while difficulty in breathing is extreme. The bloat may be frothy in type, when salivation is common in addition to the other symptoms.

TREATMENT. If discovered in time the following remedies will be of use.
1. *Antimonium Crudum 6c.* Useful in frothy bloat which comes on quickly after eating. Dose: one every hour for four doses.
2. *Apis Mellifica 6c.* This remedy will help control the amount of fluid generated in frothy bloat. Dose: one every half-hour for four doses.
3. *Carbo Vegetabilis 6c.* This is suitable for less acute cases. The animal show signs of impending toxaemia. Dose: one every hour for four doses.
4. *Colchicum 6c.* More acute cases if seen in time will respond to this remedy. Dose: one every half-hour for six doses.

9. Abscess of Liver. This may arise as a sequel to ulceration of some part of the upper digestive tract. A bacterial cause is fusiformis leading to abscess formation in a portion of damaged liver parenchyma. Any septic condition producing metastases may contribute to the formation of liver abscess.

SYMPTOMS. These are frequently indefinite but are usually those associated with peritonitis. The liver may be enlarged in which case it can be felt through the fossa posterior to the last rib.

TREATMENT. Any treatment offered is designed to ameliorate the general condition and reduce toxaemia, enabling an animal to be prepared for salvage. The judicious use of certain remedies may enable a particularly valuable animal to be saved.
1. *Hepar Sulph 200c. or 1m.* The higher potencies of this remedy will help resolve abscesses and prevent toxic complications. Dose: one night and morning for ten days.
2. *Mercuris Dulcis 30c.* This is a good general liver remedy and has proved valuable in the treatment of various conditions affecting this gland. Dose: one three times daily for two weeks.
3. *Silicea 200c.* Will aid absorption of scar tissue in the liver which may be associated with abscess formation. Will help the abscess to resolve. Dose: one daily for ten days.

10. Necrotic Hepatitis. Inflammation of liver associated with necrotic areas in the liver parenchyma.

ETIOLOGY. This is bacterial, *Fusiformis necrophorus* being the main cause.

SYMPTOMS. This condition is more common in animals under three years old than in older ones. A high temperature accompanies an arched back, stiffness and grunting, signs associated with peritonitis. Jaundice has occasionally been seen but is uncommon. Respirations are greatly increased. Pain between the last two ribs on the right-hand side, revealed by percussion, and associated with liver enlargement, suggests this condition.

TREATMENT.
1. *Kali Carbonicum 30c.* Associated with dropsy and pain worse on *left* side. Dose: one three times daily for four days.
2. *Phosphorus 200c.* This remedy is associated with degeneration of liver tissue. Controls the tendency to secondary abscess formation. Dose: one daily for one week.
3. *Silecea 200c.* Will help resolution and aid resorption of dead tissue. Dose: one dose daily for ten days.

4. Diseases of the Nervous System

1. Meningitis. This is usually secondary to some bacterial or viral condition, but a primary form can occasionally occur.

ETIOLOGY. The commoner secondary form arises as a result of spread within the body from some generalised condition. It may take a purulent or haemorrhagic form, the former being associated with pyogenic infections, e.g. navel-ill in calves, metritis in cows, etc. Metallic poisonings can lead to haemorrhagic meningitis.

SYMPTOMS. There is an early rise in temperature in most cases. Restlessness and head shaking are common which can go on to pressing the head against any suitable object. These symptoms may be followed by periods of depression. Muscular twitchings and spasms may appear, the favourite area being the neck region, but also occuring on the flank. Retraction of the head is a common symptom.

TREATMENT.
1. *Aconite 6c.* The early feverish state will be controlled by this remedy and its use will sometimes prevent more serious symptoms developing. Dose: one every half-hour for six doses.
2. *Apis Mellifica 6c.* The acute form is sometimes associated with oedema of the meninges and this remedy will benefit such cases. Dose: one every half-hour for five doses.
3. *Belladonna 1m.* Excitement and cerebral involvement call for this. Frequent head shakings occur. Dose: one every hour for four doses.
4. *Cicuta Virosa 200c.* Indicated in twitching of neck muscles with contraction and drawing back of head which may be twisted to one side. Dose: one twice daily for five days.
5. *Zincum Metallicum 30c.* Head shaking and rolling call for this remedy when there is an accompanying paddling of feet. Dose: one twice daily for six days.

2. Cerebral Oedema. This condition sometimes accompanies brain disease of ruminants.

ETIOLOGY.   Encephalomalacia is the commonest cause but it can also arise as a result of brain injury.

CLINICAL FINDINGS.   Blindness is an early symptom. Convulsions and muscle tremors occur, along with opisthotonus. Muscle incoordination soon sets in and the animal may become recumbent with increased convulsions.

TREATMENT.
1. *Apis Mellifica 6c.*   This is the remedy of choice in oedematous states. Dose: one three times daily for three days.
2. *Belladonna 1m.*   Excitement and convulsions should be allayed by this remedy. Dose: one every hour for four doses.
3. *Cicuta Virosa 200c.*   Neck twitchings and blindness indicate the possibility of this remedy helping the condition. Squinting of the eyes is a prominent sign. Dose: one night and morning for four days.
4. *Strychninum 200c.*   Indicated in opisthotonus, muscle rigidity and twitchings. Dose: one three times daily for four days.

3. Encephalitis. Inflammation of the brain. This is not uncommon in cattle of all age groups.

ETIOLOGY.   Most cases of encephalitis are related to bacterial or viral infection.

SYMPTOMS.   There is early fever, dependent on invasion by the causal organism. The heart rate is increased and dullness and lack of appetite appear. Excitement may be an early sign. Brain involvement is evident by bellowing, head shaking and staring pupils. This may lead on to head pressing, convulsions and champing of jaws. Muscle tremors appear on the limbs and face. Unsteadiness of gait is common and may lead to paralysis.

TREATMENT.
1. *Aconite 6c.*   The early feverish state calls for this remedy. Dose: one every hour for four hours.

2. *Belladonna 1m.* For convulsions, excitement and head pressing. The pupils are dilated as a rule. Dose: one hourly for four doses.
3. *Cuprum 30c.* Muscle tremors, cramps and rigidity may be helped by Cuprum. Dose: one daily for four days.
4. *Hyoscyamus 200c.* Frequent head shaking calls for this remedy. There is also a tendency to muscular twitchings. Dose: one three times daily for four days.
5. *Stramonium 30c.* Indicated in vertigo with a tendency to stagger and fall sideways. Dose: one twice daily for one week.

5. Affections of the Musculo-skeletal System

1. Gonitis. This is an inflammation of the stifle joint and is not uncommon in cattle. When occurring in bulls it seriously interferes with service. It is invariably sub-acute or chronic.

ETIOLOGY. It frequently arises as a sequel to some severe sprain. Old animals are involved as result of joint degeneration.

SYMPTOMS. A shortened stride is seen on the affected side. Flexion of joints occurs. Extension of the joint in movement produces pain. The joint is obviously enlarged in severe cases while less severe involvement can be deduced by palpation of the joint.

TREATMENT.
1. *Arnica 30c.* This should always be given if injury is suspected as a contributory cause. Dose: two doses 24 hours apart.
2. *Rhus Toxicodendron 1m.* When sprain has been implicated to begin with. Dose: one daily for one week.
3. *Ruta Graveolens 30c.* If the periosteum of the bone is suspected of involvement. Dose: one twice daily for one week.
4. *Symphytum 200c.* Surface fracture of a bone at the time of the original injury will benefit from this remedy. Dose: one daily for one week.

1. Osteodystrophy. This term signifies a disturbance of normal bone development. Developed bone may also be involved when abnormal growth takes place. Rickets in young animals and osteomalacia in older ones are manifestations of it.

ETIOLOGY. These disturbances and changes are usually due to deficiencies of calcium, phosphorus and Vitamin D, or to change in the normal CA : P ratio.

SYMPTOMS. Distortion and enlargement of bones accompany a susceptibility to fracture. Normal movement is interfered with. Weakening of bones leads to fractures and deformities depending on the age of the animal. Bony enlargements may occur at the ends of long bones.

TREATMENT.
1. *Calcium Phosphate 30c.* Young animals especially respond well to this remedy. The enlargements at the bone ends are painful. Dose: one per day for two–three weeks.
2. *Phosphoric Acid 30c.* This is another useful remedy for young animals, especially rapidly growing dairy calves. Dose: one daily for two weeks.

3. Abscess of the Foot. This is not an uncommon condition among animals kept in unsanitary conditions.

ETIOLOGY. Injury can play a prominent part, penetrating wounds of the sole being a common cause.

SYMPTOMS. Lameness due to severe pain is the first sign that something is wrong. The foot is usually held raised off the ground. Occasionally a sinus develops when the pain becomes less severe.

TREATMENT.
1. *Aconite 6c.* If seen early this remedy will ease pain and settle the animal. Dose: one every hour for four doses.
2. *Hepar Sulphuricum 30c.* In the acute stage, this potency will help the abscess to resolve. Lower potencies may help drainage of purulent material. Dose: one every two hours for four doses.
3. *Silicia 200c.* Useful in the more chronic form. Will help dry up the sinuses which may develop. Dose: one per day for ten days.

4. Foul in the Foot – Foot Rot. This is an infection of the foot which leads to interdigital dermatitis and necrosis, with, in neglected cases, secondary infection extending as far as the pastern joint.

ETIOLOGY. The bacterium *Fusiformis necrophorus* is the main organism concerned, while pyogenic bacteria are responsible for secondary infection.

SYMPTOMS. Necrosis of the interdigital space usually follows a dermatitis beginning at the centre of the coronary band between the digits. Lameness is usually severe and the characteristic smell of necrotic tissue is present. Secondary invasion by pyogenic bacteria leads to swelling of tissues as far as the pastern joint, while an arthritis may develop in the joint itself.

TREATMENT.
1. *Calcarea Fluorica 30c.* Will help control pedal ostitis and prevent tissue overgrowth. Dose: one per day for seven days.
2. *Hepar Sulphuricum 30c.* Secondary infection in the acute stage will be helped by this remedy. Dose: one three times daily for two days.
3. *Natrum Muriaticum 200c.* This remedy has a useful role to play in foot conditions of this nature. Dose: one per day for ten days.
4. *Silicea 200c.* More especially for chronic states. Will control the necrosis of tissue and clear the foot of purulent material. Dose: one per day for ten days.

5. Laminitis. Overfeeding can cause this condition, producing disturbances in the foot and leading to distortion of hooves.

ETIOLOGY. Engorging on concentrates is the primary cause. The condition can arise if beef animals are introduced to rich feeding too suddenly. Show animals are frequently at risk.

SYMPTOMS. Disturbances of digestion first appear followed by a slow or stilted walk. Later the hooves become elongated and grooved.

TREATMENT.
1. *Aconite 6x.* When foot symptoms appear due to inflammation of inner structures. Dose: one half-hourly for six doses.
2. *Belladonna 1m.* This remedy can safely be alternated with aconite in acute cases. Dose: one every half-hour for six doses.
3. *Calcarea Fluorica 30c.* Once the hoof becomes elongated and grooved. Dose: one daily for one week followed by one monthly for 3 months.
4. *Nux Vomica 200c.* This remedy will help the initial digestive upset. Dose: one three times daily for two days.

1. Interdigital Hyperplasia. This is a foot affection which occurs as an overgrowth of connective tissue between the digits. The protrusions are referred to as corns, and can become the seat of necrotic infection.

ETIOLOGY. Long-standing irritation is the main cause, often due to faulty conformation or infection due to *Fusiformis necrophorus.*

SYMPTOMS. Lameness can occur and the animal walks in a stilted manner. The protrusions are obvious as swellings between digits. Secondary infection may lead to swelling above the coronary band.

TREATMENT.
1. *Calcarea Fluorica 30c.* This remedy will prevent the development of further growth and acts generally as a good tissue remedy. Dose: one per week for one month.
2. *Silicea 200c.* The main remedy for reducing existing excess tissue. It has beneficial action on the foot generally and aids the absorption of scar tissue. Dose: one daily for two weeks.
3. *Natrum Muriaticum 200c.* Necrotic infection and ulcerations will be helped by this remedy. Dose: one daily for one week.

6. Diseases of the Urinary System

1. Acute Nephritis. Inflammation of the kidney substance is rarely a primary condition.

ETIOLOGY. Septicaemic infections are a principle cause and it may also arise as a sequel to mastitis, metritis or some other septic condition. Poisoning by chemical mineral and plant agents frequently leads to nephritis.

SYMPTOMS. Initial rise of temperature is followed by anorexia and possibly increased respiration. Tenderness over the kidney area is common. Frequent urination of small amounts of highly-coloured urine is attended with occasional difficulty in passing. The urine itself may contain blood, pus and mucus. Albuminuria is present.

TREATMENT.
1. *Aconite 30c.* An essential remedy in the early feverish stage, especially when associated with a primary infectious condition. Dose: one every hour for four doses.
2. *Apis Mellifica 6c.* The early acute stage is usually attended by oedematous infiltration of tissue and Apis is a useful remedy in this connection. Dose: one every half-hour for six doses.
3. *Arsenicum Album 1m.* Indicated when there is scanty albuminous urine showing shreds of mucus. Thirst for small quantities is a prominent sign. Dose: one every three hours for four doses.
4. *Berberis Vulgaris 6c.* Tenderness over the kidneys and sacral region accompanies frequent urination. the urine is cloudy and contains a reddish sediment. Dose: one dose three hourly for four doses.
5. *Terebinthinae 200c.* Scanty blood-stained urine. Difficulty in passing. Sweetish odour. Frequently associated with infections. Dose: one twice daily for three days.
6. *Uva Ursi 3x.* The urine may contain bile and pus along with clotted blood and mucus. Dose: one thrice daily for four days.

2. Purulent Nephritis – Abscess of Kidney.

ETIOLOGY. This usually accompanies any acute or chronic septic condition which results in metastatic spread to the kidney via the blood-stream. This may be seen in navel-ill of calves or septic mastitis.

SYMPTOMS. Emaciation follows long spells of indifferent feeding. Urine examination may show the presence of pus.

TREATMENT. This is purely related to the value of the animal. The following remedies may enable the owner to prepare an animal for salvage or possibly to save a more valuable animal.
1. *Hepar Sulph 1m.* Higher potencies of this remedy will help control the original septic state and produce an improvement in the general health. Dose: one every two hours for four doses. Should be followed later by higher potencies if improvement results.
2. *Silicea 200c.* If chronic liver or lung abscess is suspected as a contributory cause, this remedy may help. Dose: one daily for ten days.

3. Pyelonephritis. This infection of the kidney is the commonest urinary tract affection of cattle.

ETIOLOGY. A specific organism of the corynebacteria is usually associated with this condition. A latent state may be aggravated by dystokia or infection arising from parturition.

SYMPTOMS. A muco-purulent discharge may be seen following a difficult calving due to an extension of infection from the uterus. Loss of condition rapidly follows. Symptoms of colic sometimes appear when the animal kicks at the belly and may stretch out the hind-legs. Frequent straining accompanies blood-stained urine containing pus.

TREATMENT.
1. *Benzoicum Acidum 6c.* Cases resembling cystitis will do well on this remedy. The urine is strong smelling and contains catarrhal deposits. Dose: one three times daily for five days.

2. *Hepar Sulphuricum 200c.* There may be tenderness over the loins when this remedy is needed. More suitable for the acute case. Dose: one every two hours for four doses.
3. *Mercurius Corrosivus 200c.* Slimy blood-stained urine containing mucus shreds and pus indicates this remedy. Dose: one three times daily for three days.
4. *Silicea 200c.* Suitable for the more chronic case. The pus when present is whitish-grey in colour. Dose: one dose daily for ten days.

4. Cystitis. Inflammation of the bladder may be primary or secondary, the latter being the more common, and may also be acute or chronic.

ETIOLOGY. The acute form is usually bacterial in origin, while the chronic form may be associated with gravel or sand in the urine.

SYMPTOMS. Frequent urination is the commonest sign, the urine containing blood. There may be considerable difficulty in passing urine. Arching of the back and signs of pain are evident, such as kicking at abdomen.

TREATMENT.
1. *Cantharis 6c.* Scanty amounts of blood-stained urine with straining. Signs of abdominal pain prominent. Dose: one every two hours for four doses.
2. *Copaiva 6c.* Catarrhal cystitis with increase of mucus in urine, which has a sweetish smell. Dose: one every two hours for four doses.
3. *Cubebs 6c.* Another useful remedy to remember in cases of profuse muco-purulent urination. There is increased urination but less strangury than with cantharis. Dose: one three times daily for four doses.
4. *Thlaspi Bursa 6c.* Chronic states are well served by this remedy. Gravelly or sandy deposits are common in the urine. Dose: one three times daily for seven days.
5. *Uva Ursi 3x.* Also useful in chronic cystitis. Urine is slimy. Pain and straining common. Dose: one three times daily for seven days.

7. Affections of the Skin

1. Photosensitisation. This is a sensitivity to strong sunlight affecting unpigmented areas of skin.

ETIOLOGY. It is frequently associated with the ingestion of certain plants; e.g. St. John's Wort (Hypericum).

SYMPTOMS. A dermatitis first appears on the unpigmented areas of the skin which eventually become necrosed. Oozing of serum and swelling accompany the dermatitis. Lesions may be seen around the eyes, muzzle, teats and along the back. Internal derangement is manifested by jaundice. This icteric form may be accompanied by lachrymation, salivation and diarrhoea. Itching and head shaking occur. The muzzle assumes a coppery appearance.

TREATMENT.
1. *Arenicum Album 30c.* A useful general skin remedy. Will help promote new growth of hair. Dose: one daily for ten days.
2. *Chelidonium 30c.* A useful remedy for icteric cases. Dose: one twice daily for seven days.
3. *Hypericum 6c.* Will help counteract the effects of ingestion of St. John's Wort. Will also relieve pain in nerve endings. Dose: one twice daily for five days.
4. *Rhus Toxicodendron 1m.* This remedy will help in the early acute stage associated with inflammation and oozing of serum. Dose: one three hourly for four doses.
5. *Sulphur 6x.* Redness, swelling and itching will benefit from sulphur. Dose: one three times daily for three days.

2. Ringworm. This is a superficial fungus disease of the skin and is more common in the younger age group.

ETIOLOGY. Various species of fungi are incriminated.

SYMPTOMS.   The lesions usually assume a circular appearance and in severe cases may be large and extensive. The skin becomes dry and scaly and scurfy. Itching is considerable. The head and neck are favourite sites. The crusts on the lesions may be hard and scab-like.

TREATMENT.
1. *Bacillinum 200c.*   This nosode is probably the most effective remedy. Dose: one only, repeated in one month.
2. *Kali Arsenicum 200c.*   A useful remedy to restore condition to the skin after bacillinum has produced a cure. Dose: one daily for seven days.
3. *Tellurium 6c.*   This remedy will also prove useful in growing hair over affected areas. An indication for its use is the formation of circular lesions, more especially around ears. Dose: one daily for seven days.

3.   Mange.   Sometimes called scabies or itch. The three main types are Psoroptic, Sarcoptic and Chorioptic.

a. *Psoroptic.*   This is highly contagious and confined to cattle. It may be spread by direct contact or through the medium of contaminated bedding, etc.

SYMPTOMS.   Psoroptic – Lesions usually begin on the shoulders and dorsal area of the neck. Localised inflammation from the bites of the mites produces intense itching. Lesions become papular and ooze serum. This exudation mats the hair and produces a scab in due course, each scab tending to enlarge and coalesce with others. The mites remain on the skin surface.

b. *Sarcoptic.*   In this form the mites burrow under the skin, producing tunnels.

SYMPTOMS Sarcoptic – Areas of swelling and inflammation accompany the burrowing process. Itching is severe. Rubbing the skin leads to bare patches and in prolonged or neglected cases to thickening of the skin which becomes wrinkled into folds.

c. *Chorioptic.*   Sometimes called Symbiotic or tail mange. This is usually mild and confined to cattle.

SYMPTOMS.   Chorioptic – Lesions remain small and are confined to tail and legs. Itching is present but is not severe.

TREATMENT. The following remedies will assist the action of external dressings and dips and are not intended as a substitute.

1. *Sulphur 30c.* This is a good general remedy which will produce a body climate unfavourable to mites. Dose: one daily for seven days.
2. *Psorinum 30c.* A useful remedy which will help control severe itch. More for dry skins. Dose: one daily for seven days.
3. *Kali Arsenicum 200c.* When the skin is thrown into thick wrinkled folds. Scurf is abundant. Dose: one daily for ten days.

8. Bracken Poisoning

This may be acute or sub-acute

ETIOLOGY. It is due to a toxic principle found in bracken and ingested when the fronds are green and succulent. Poisoning occurs mainly after a drought when normal grazing becomes scarce. Contamination of grazing by rabbits has caused animals to eat bracken. The effects are cumulative and toxic symptoms may not appear until a few weeks have passed after consumption.

SYMPTOMS. The temperature is very high and may reach 107–108°F. Depression and anorexia occur: faeces become loose and watery, and contain flecks of blood or more frank bleeding. There may be difficulty in breathing when laryngeal oedema occurs. Small haemorrhages occur on the visible mucosae.

TREATMENT. The following remedies may prove beneficial in the milder cases and are worth trying:
1. *Crotalus Horridus 200c.* This is an excellent remedy for controlling internal bleeding generally. Indicated in passive haemorrhage, the blood usually being dark. Dose: one every hour for four doses, followed by one twice daily. Higher potencies should be tried on more acute cases.
2. *Ipecacuanha 30c.* A useful remedy when the haemorrhages are of bright red blood. Nasal bleeding is often present when this remedy is indicated. Dose: one four times in 24 hours followed by one twice daily for three days.
3. *Phosphorus 1m.* Petechial haemorrhages on the mucosae in the milder case may be helped by this remedy. Dose: one dose three times daily for three days.
4. *Ficus Religiosa 6c.* A good remedy for controlling haemorrhages generally. Respiratory distress is often present. Dose: one three times daily for five days.

9. Sweet Clover Poisoning

This is a haemorrhagic condition causing anaemia and death in severe cases.

ETIOLOGY. Ingestion of white Sweet Clover (Melilotus spp) causing release of dicoumarin, the toxic principle which is formed during spoiling of the clover crop. Signs of poisoning may suddenly appear if an animal is subjected to surgical interference during the build-up of a toxic state.

SYMPTOMS. There is paleness of visible mucous membranes. Stiffness, dullness and loss of condition are evident. The heart rate is increased if much blood is lost. Nose-bleeding may occur. Haematomatous swellings may appear anywhere on the body.

TREATMENT. In slow, less acute cases the following remedies may be found useful:
1. *Crotalus Horridus 200c.* A very good anti-haemorrhagic remedy, especially from small visceral blood-vessels. Blood may be dark. Dose: one four times daily for one day. Follow with one night and morning of 30c.
2. *Ferrum Phosphoricum 6c.* Indicated when there is accompanying stiffness and possibly bleeding from the lungs. The temperature may be raised. Dose: one four times in 24 hours.
3. *Ipecacuanha 30c.* When the blood is bright red and there is a tendency to nose-bleeding. Faeces may be loose. Dose: one every three hours for four doses.
4. *Millefolium 30c.* The blood is also bright red when this remedy is indicated. Bleeding frequently occurs from the uterus and blood may be seen in the urine. Dose: one three times daily for three days.
5. *Sabina 6c.* Bright red blood which does not clot readily. Uterine and kidney haemorrhaging prominent. Dose: one every 24 hours for four doses.

10. Mineral Deficiencies

In my experience the question of trace element deficiency does not arise on farms which are run on organic lines, but it is a frequent cause of unthriftiness of stock grazing on deficient pastures, or on those which have been over-fertilised with inorganic manures. The elements we are here considering are calcium, magnesium, phosphorus, sodium and potassium, together with cobalt and copper. In many soils these first five elements are present in the wrong proportion, and it has been proved that each must have the proper ratio to the other before the animal can make correct use of them. In a healthy organic soil this balance in maintained by soil bacteria, but where the balance is distorted and the ratio upset, diseases like hypomagnesaemia and aphosphorosis may assume serious proportions, while milk fever could become an additional hazard at parturition. Where strict organic husbandry is not possible these trace element deficiencies can best be controlled by the use of homoeopathic remedies incorporating the remedies in combination, such as Calcarea Phosphorica and Magnesium Phosphoricum together with various Kali (potassium) and Natrum (Sodium) salts. If, for example, in-calf cows were given a course of Calc. Phos. weekly for the last trimester of pregnancy, it would greatly reduce the likelihood of milk fever or grass tetany arising. Supplying these elements in homoeopathic potentised form provides the surest way of having them retained in the system. Otherwise, they are quickly excreted.

Mineral Deficiencies and Disorders of Metabolism

1. Calcium and Phosphorus. Phosphorus deficiency – aphosphorosis – is frequently found and is commonly associated with a disturbed Ca : P ratio. Soils deficient in phosphorus will obviously be unbalanced as regards the ratio of one trace element to another.

SYMPTOMS. Calcium deficiency in the young animal may take the form of rickets, which leads to the deposition of uncalcified bone around the joints and bending of the long bones. In the adult animal this deficiency is called osteomalacia, in which normal bone is absorbed. Osteo-fibrosis also arises.

Phosphorus deficiency may also lead to depraved appetite – Pica – such as eating strange objects, e.g. bones or leather. Deficiency may also show in sub-fertility, probably because of ovarian dysfunction.

Roughage of poor quality may lead to calcium deficiency, or when feed is grown on soils deficient in the mineral.

TREATMENT.
1. *Calcarea Phosphorica 30c.*   This is the remedy of choice in both Ca and P deficiencies, and should be given as a routine remedy to all young stock during the first three months, one dose per week being adequate. This will do much to prevent acute cases arising. For treatment in the acute case, one dose per day for two weeks should suffice.

   It must be understood that this remedy should supplement a diet containing adequate vitamins and other trace elements.

2.   Magnesium Deficiency – Grass Tetany.   This condition usually occurs in early summer when animals are grazed on heavily fertilised ground, and also in the autumn, particularly in wet weather, after overnight frosts. It occurs mainly in the cow which has calved a few weeks previously, and is milking heavily. Attacks can be sudden and severe, although milder forms also occur. Sudden deaths are the result of a hyper-acute form.

SYMPTOMS.   Clonic and tonic spasms are present in mild cases, and the animal is seen to tremble. Such cases can develop into the acute form when brain involvement occurs, leading to convulsions and eventual coma. There are little if any prodromal signs associated with the hyper-acute forms and susceptible animals can drop dead within a minute or two of the condition developing.

TREATMENT.   While calcium and magnesium injections are recognised as the standard treatment, the following remedies will help recovery and limit any damage to the central nervous system.
1. *Cuprum Aceticum 6c.*   A useful remedy for the milder case which comes on suddenly and is associated with cramps and spasms with a paralytic tendency. If given early it may well pre-

vent the onset of convulsions and cut short an acute attack. The limbs appear to be shuddering, but coldness is absent. Dose: one every three hours for five doses.

2. *Belladonna 1m.*   Probably the most useful remedy for the acute attack presented with convulsions, dilated pupils and general brain involvement. Dose: one every half-hour for six doses.

3. *Stramonium 200c.*   With this remedy the animal is usually standing, but showing a tendency to fall forward to the left side. If the animal is on the ground there is a raising and lowering of the head. Dose: one every two hours for four doses.

4. *Cicuta Virosa 200c.*   Somewhat similar to the previous remedy, but in this case the neck shows a distinct twist or backward inclination. Muscles of head and neck may show twitching. Dose: one every hour for four doses.

5. *Magnesium Phosphoricum 30c.*   This remedy should be given along with the selected remedy, one dose alternating with the other for four doses.

In all cases, the animal; should be kept as quiet as possible, and protected from bright light and sudden noise. Even mild cases have been known to react adversely to sudden frights and noises. In-calf cows should be given Mag. Phos. 30c in weekly doses for the two months preceding calving, and before the advent of the spring grass. This remedy may with advantage be combined with Kali. Phos. 30c as it is considered likely that the element potassium is implicated in the development of attacks.

3.   Transport Tetany.   This is a form of hypocalcaemia sometimes observed in transported animals. Cows of five years old and upwards are chiefly affected, and of this class, the animal in the last trimester of pregnancy is most at risk. The danger of an attack is less likely in the freshly calved cow.

ETIOLOGY.   It is thought to be due to a disorder of the calcium metabolism.

CLINICAL SIGNS.   Early symptoms include ataxia and restlessness, which leads to partial paralysis of the hind-quarters, with muscular spasms, and stiffness. Hyper-excitability is a common feature, and sometimes accompanies foaming at the mouth. The animal may stagger and fall down. Respirations are increased, while digestive symptoms include lack of appetite, and cessation of rumenation. A comatose form may supervene in the later stages.

TREATMENT. The standard calcium injections should be supplemented by one or other of the following remedies according to symptoms shown.
1. *Belladonna 1m.* When hyper-excitability is the main feature, the cow showing dilated pupils and a full bounding pulse. Dose: one every half-hour for four doses.
2. *Cuprum Metallicum 1m.* For muscular spasms and stiffness. Dose: one three times daily for two days.
3. *Agaricus Muscarius 30c.* When ataxia is prominent, the animal showing a tendency to fall forward. Dose: one every three hours for four doses.
4. *Opium 200c.* A useful remedy for the comatose state. The animal lies perfectly still, often with the head turned towards the flank. Dose: one dose.
5. *Calcium Phos. 30c and Magnesium Phos. 30c.* The combination of these two remedies will help stabilise the calcium and magnesium metabolism, and prevent relapse. Dose: one three times daily for two days.

4. Milk Fever. Parturient Hypocalcaemia. Parturient Paresis. This is one of the lactation diseases commonly seen in cows which have attained their highest productive period.

ETIOLOGY. The immediate cause is a reduction or fall in the level of calcium in the system. This is brought about by too little calcium being fed, together with the demands made on the dam's reserves by the developing foetus, and finally by the further drain on the calcium reserves by the onset of lactation.

SYMPTOMS. The average attack takes place within 72 hours after parturition, but cases may occur before the calf is born, and, exceptionally, it may occur later in the lactation period. Preliminary signs include ataxia and restlessness, these signs becoming more severe until the animal becomes wobbly and finally collapses. Coma may or may not set in, but when it does, a common pose is that of the animal lying recumbent with the head turned round to one side, resting on the neck. Occasionally the neck assumes a lateral or S curve. Just as frequent is the patient lying stretched out and groaning. Muscular tremors may be seen. Tympany sets in if the animal has collapsed with the rumen uppermost. Congestion of the eye is usually present. Temperature is invariably sub-normal.

TREATMENT. The classical treatment of this disease is by intravenous or subcutaneous injection of calcium and allied salts, and in the great majority of cases this is successful, no other treatment being needed. The disease is included in this work because the addition of selected homoepathic remedies to the orthodox injections will greatly reduce the risk of relapse, and help prevent complications of the nervous system. These remedies include the following:

1. *Belladonna 1m.* This is indicated when the animal is excitable or violent, throwing the head about, with staring pupils and congested eyes. Dose: one every half hour for four doses.

2. *Magnesium Phosphoricum 6c.* Should always be given as a routine, to obviate the danger of magnesium deficiency co-existing with the calcium. Dose: one every hour for four doses.

3. *Stramonium 200c.* When nervous symptoms are more often seen on peripheral parts, with less brain involvement. Twitchings are commonly seen. Dose: one every hour for six doses.

4. *Opium 200c.* A useful remedy for the comatose patient which lies still, with stertorous breathing. Dose: two doses two hours apart.

5. *Thyroid 3x.* The administration of this remedy will help regulate thyroid function, this gland being deeply involved in the disease process. Dose: one every hour for 3 doses, followed by one thrice daily for two days.

6. *Cuprum Metallicum 1m.* This remedy will assist in relieving subsequent muscular cramping when the animal is on the way to recovery. Dose: one twice daily for two days.

7. *Colchicum 200c.* If rumenal bloat is a problem, the administration of this remedy every half-hour for four doses will relieve.

Prevention of milk fever. The weekly adminstration of Calc. Phos. 30c and Magnesium Phos. 30c will help the cow to retain normal mineral reserves. This is difficult to achieve by conventional means, as these elements are excreted quickly in the crude form. The homoeopathic potentised remedy possesses the property of being assimilated properly. Treatment should cover the last three months of pregnancy.

5. Acetonaemia. Ketosis. This is a metabolic disease which can occur in lactating animals up to six weeks or two months after calving. It can affect first calvers as well as older animals.

ETIOLOGY. Carbohydrate deficiency is believed to play a part, resulting in a lowering of circulating glucose in the blood. Also implicated is a disturbance of the adrenal gland function.

SYMPTOMS. A great variety of clinical signs exists, but broadly speaking there are nervous and digestive forms, each producing its own clinical picture. The nervous form is manifested by extreme nervousness and excitability. Stalled animals may exhibit climbing movements with frequent head-shaking, which may end in convulsions. Occasionally a comatose state is seen. Digestive forms show inappetance with a sharp drop in milk production. Loss of condition rapidly supervenes. Occasionally appetite is maintained, but only for certain types of food. The abdomen is tucked up and rumenal sounds and movements are in abeyance. Grinding of teeth may be heard, and the dung is dry and glazed-looking. The sweet smell of acidosis may be detected on the breath and in the milk, but this is not a constant sign.

TREATMENT. This varies according to whether nervous or digestive symptoms predominate.
1. *Aconitum 12x.* This remedy may alleviate nervous signs if given early. It is a valuable remedy for bringing about a state of calm. Dose: one every hour for three dose.
2. *Stramonium 200c.* Useful for controlling the tendency to fits or convulsions. Dose: one every hour for four doses.
3. *Cicuta Virosa 6c.* Also valuable for some forms of nervous upsets. The patient usually has a staring look, and the head may appear twisted round due to deviation of neck muscles. Dose: one every two hours for four doses.
4. *Opium 200c.* If comatose forms arise with the patient in a collapsed, sleepy state. Dose: two doses two hours apart.
5. *Lycopodium 1m.* This is the main remedy in the digestive form. It produces a tonic action on the liver, regulating the gylycogen

function and restoring normal glucose levels in the blood. Dose: one per day for ten days.

6. *Nux Vomica 1m.* A valuable remedy for restoring normal digestion. Should be given after Lycopodium. Dose: one daily for five days.

6. Cobalt Deficiency. Sometimes referred to as cobalt pine, this condition is confined to certain areas, and is associated with a state of inappetance in the older animals, suckling calves not being affected.

CLINICAL SIGNS. These consist of general unthriftiness, dry harsh coat, stunted growth, and lachrymation. Occasionally grinding of the teeth suggests digestive disturbance and accompanies lack of rumenation and anorexia. Signs of anaemia are invariably present, e.g. pallor of visible mucous membranes. Dandruff scales are often present in the coat.

TREATMENT. Cobalt given in the form of the potentised (1m) metal or its chloride will help stabilise the element in the system and is useful as long-term therapy after admininstration of cobalt solutions and/or vitamin B12 in the short-term. Dose: Cobaltum 1m and Cobaltum Chloridum 30c – one dose per week for three months.

7. Iron Deficiency. This condition often co-exists with cobalt deficiency, but may be met with as a separate entity.

CLINICAL SIGNS. These include loss of appetite, emaciation, weakness and anaemia. Blood examination shows a significant lowering of the haemoglobin content.

TREATMENT.
1. *Ferrum Metallicum 6x.* In the potentised form the animal's system will respond better to medication than iron given in the conventional manner, when frequently the body is unable to utilise it properly. Dose: one three times daily for two weeks.
2. *Ferrum Iodatum 6c.* Respiratory symptoms such as mucous discharges from the lungs sometimes containing blood are pre-

sent when this remedy is indicated. Dose: one three times daily for one week.

3. *Ferrum Muriaticum 6c.* Heart symptoms are prominent, such as weak thready pulse and rapid breathing on exercise. There may be evidence of internal haemorrhage such as the presence of blood in the urine. Dose: one three times daily for one week.

4. *Cinchona 6c.* A very useful remedy to combat the weakness associated with the anaemia which arises. Dose: one twice daily for two weeks.

5. *Natrum Muriaticum 30c.* This is a good remedy for longer-term administration. It helps regulate the salt metabolism and stabilises fluid elimination. Dose: one per day for two weeks.

6. *Trinitrotoluene 30c.* Muscular cramps and jaundice are additional signs to those already mentioned under other remedies. It has particularly favourable effect on haemoglobin, helping it to perform its function more effectively. Dose: one three times daily for one week.

11. Protozoal Diseases

1. Redwater or Babesiasis. This disease is characterised by high temperature and destruction of red cells leading to anaemia and haemoglobinuria.

ETIOLOGY. Various species of Babesia are involved, this being a protozoon organism transmitted by ticks.

SYMPTOMS. The incubation period is up to three weeks. The temperature thereafter rises quickly – up to 105°F or 106°F – and is accompanied by lack of appetite, depression and cessation of milk yield. The heart rate is increased and heart beats are audible without the aid of the stethoscope. Respirations are also increased. Anaemia is evidenced by pallor of visible mucous membranes, while the urine becomes dark red. Some species of Babesia produce an action on the anal sphincter leading to the passage of long thin ropy faeces without actual diarrhoea.

TREATMENT. Homoeopathic treatment will help supplement the standard injections which are specific for the condition. Among those which will be of use are the following:
1. *China Officinalis 6c.* Useful for restoring strength after loss of blood. Dose: one three times daily for five days.
2. *Millefolium 30c.* A valuable remedy for loss of blood generally. Dose: one three times daily for five days.
3. *Ficus Religiosa 6c.* This is also a good anti-haemorrhagic remedy especially useful when respiratory symptoms predominate. Dose: one three times daily for one week.
4. *Phosphorus 1m.* Liver involvement evidenced by jaundice sometimes sets in during the course of the disease and this remedy will then be found useful. It is also of value in controlling haemorrhage. Dose: one dose twice daily for one week.
5. *Crotalus Horridus 200c.* Should be of value in preventing further haemolysing of red cells. Will also be of use in combating jaundice and haemorrhages generally. Dose: one every three hours for four doses.

Other snake venom remedies such as Vipera and Bothrops Lanciolatus also should be remembered.

2. Anaplasmosis. This infectious disease is manifested by anaemia and jaundice but differs from Babesiasis in the absence of blood in the urine.

ETIOLOGY. A protozoon organism termed *Anaplasma marginale* which appears in the red blood cells of the host animal. Insect vectors including ticks transmit the disease from affected to susceptible animals by biting.

SYMPTOMS. There is an incubation period of 3–4 weeks. The temperature may rise to 105°F or more, followed by depression, increased respiration, inappetance and a fall in milk yield. Signs of anaemia soon appear with pallor of visible mucous membranes. Jaundice is a prominent symptom discolouration being seen in the eyes and on the skin of teats and udder. The heart rate is markedly increased and emaciation and dehydration soon supervene. Occasionally a mucopurulent nasal discharge appears with muscular trembling and increased thirst. If the animal lives through the acute stages and becomes convalescent perverted appetite is seen. Bulls which recover may become temporarily infertile.

TREATMENT.
1. *Trinitrotoluene 30c.* This is an important remedy covering many of the symptoms met with in this condition from anaemia to increased heart rate and muscular cramping. Dose: one every three hours for four doses, followed by one daily for five days.
2. *Crotalus Horridus 10m.* High potencies of this remedy are valuable in combating the acute phases of the condition. The action on the liver is important. Dose: one every two hours for four doses.
3. *China 30c.* Will help restore strength in the convalescing animal. Dose: one twice daily for ten days.
4. *Phosphorus 1m.* This remedy also has an important action on the liver helping to allay destruction of cells. It should also be of use in the convalescent stage when signs of perverted appetite appear. Dose: one per day for seven days.
5. *Phytolacca 30c.* May be helpful in restoring normal testicular function in temporarily infertile male animals. Dose: one per day for two weeks.

3. Toxoplasmosis. This is a contagious disease characterised mainly by involvement of the central nervous and respiratory symptoms.

ETIOLOGY.   A protozoon organism called *Anaplasma gondii* is the cause.

SYMPTOMS.   Acute involvement is the rule beginning with pyrexia and signs of respiratory distress such as laboured breathing. Nervous involvement leads to inability to walk properly together with hyper-excitability. This phase is superseded by lethargy. The disease is passed on to unborn calves which either die soon after birth or remain weak. Respiratory and nervous symptoms also appear in calves congenitally affected, very often in a more severe form including convulsions and muscular twitchings.

TREATMENT.   If the disease is tackled in its early stages the following remedies may help:
1. *Aconitum Napellus 12x.*   Four doses at half-hourly intervals may abort the disease process if given early.
2. *Phosphorus 1m.*   Will help respiratory changes and allay a tendency to pneumonia. Dose: one every hour for four doses.
3. *Lathyrus Sativus 200c.*   A prominent remedy for controlling nervous phenomena such as ataxia and paralytic tendency. Dose: one three times daily for two days followed by one daily for three doses.
4. *Conium 30c.*   If incoordination and weakness begin first in the hind-limbs and extend forward this remedy should be of value. Dose: one thrice daily for one week.
5. *Belladonna 1m.*   When convulsions appear with general hyper-excitability. Dose: one every half-hour for four doses.
6. *Stramonium 30c.*   Another useful remedy for nervous involvement especially for muscular twitchings of isolated muscles. Will also aid convulsions. Dose: one twice daily for one week.
7. *Cuprum 1m.*   This is an important remedy if muscular crampings and rigidity occur. Dose: one daily for one week.
8. *Strychninum 200c.*   If chorea is a pronounced symptom. Dose: one twice daily for one week.

12. Mastitis

Inflammation of the udder. In the dairy cow mastitis is a complicated condition brought about by a combination of factors, such as faulty management, bacterial infections and injuries.

ETIOLOGY. The causes of mastitis have been attributed to many infective agents, the more common ones in cattle being streptococci, staphylococci, E. Coli, corynebacteria and, less frequently, pasteurellae. Staphylococci are common where prolonged use of penicillin has produced resistant strains of streptococci. The precise role of bacteria as primary causes of mastitis has not been fully determined, but other factors which appear to be of importance are unable to produce the condition in the absence of bacteria. These factors must therefore be considered only to be predisposing.

CLINICAL SIGNS. Acute, sub-acute and chronic forms are recognised. General signs include changes in milk secretion resulting in abnormalities such as clots and changes in the size and consistency of the udder of quarters involved. There is frequently also a systematic reaction.

A. Acute form. In this form, which frequently accompanies parturition, and also, in less severe form, at drying off, the onset is usually sudden, and the condition can be recognised by swelling of the gland and changes in the milk. The swelling may take several forms, ranging from slight oedema to a hot painful enlargement. Although most often seen as a sequel to calving, this acute form can also be seen at any time during lactation.

B. Chronic form. In chronic mastitis, feverish manifestations are usually absent, although exacerbations can occur. The gland shows fibrous induration in the region of the milk cistern and the milk itself shows small clots.

Mastitis caused by streptococci. In dairy herds where good hygiene and management are poorly practised, streptococci may show a morbidity rate of 25%. It is less common in well-managed herds, but can still cause a high loss of production, though rarely resulting in the death of the animal. There is a primary fever which may persist for 24 hours, but this systemic reaction is invariably mild, and is associated mainly with Streptococcus agalacticae. Streptococcus dysgalacticae and Streptococcus uberis produce a more acute syndrome with severe swelling of quarters and abnormality of milk. Systemic reaction is usually moderate, although an occasional per-acute infection may yield a very high fever.

Mastitis caused by Staphylococci.   There is frequently a per-acute form appearing a few days after parturition, and this can be highly fatal, the quarter becoming swollen and purple, and systemic involvement rapid. The chronic form of this type is characterised by a slowly developing induration of udder tissue with watery secretion, leading eventually to atrophy of the quarter. A form in between the per-acute and the chronic may yield secretion of a purulent nature containing many thick clots.

Mastitis caused by E. Coli.   Per-acute involvement is fairly common and can lead to loss of function of affected quarters and in many cases to death. The secretion is thin and yellow, and contains small bran-like flakes. Temperature may be very high indicating a severe systemic involvement.

Mastitis caused by Corynebacterium pyogenes.   This is usually called summer mastitis because of its appearance during the summer months among animals that are not lactating. In Britain it is common in warm wet summers, although it can occur under other conditions also. Low-lying wooded farms experience a high incidence and this has led some authorities to implicate flies in its transmission. Summer mastitis always commences acutely with severe systemic reaction. The quarter or quarters involved – there are frequently more than one – become indurated, yielding a thick cheese-like secretion which is evil-smelling and sometimes difficult to express. Less severe involvement produces a purulent discharge. The udder may later show abscesses which burst through the outer skin, yielding a creamy pus with occasional sloughing of tissue. The corynebacteria are well-known for the invasive toxins they produce, and it is this toxin which produces the systemic symptoms.

The role of Homoeopathy in mastitis control.

(a) *Prevention.*   When advising the dairy farmer with this end in view, we stress the importance of tackling the problem on a herd basis, rather than seeking out one or two offending animals and treating them individually as is often done by farmers themselves. In considering prevention we must take account of the various bacteriological causes of the condition, and, if possible, employ the appropriate nosode. By first determining which type of mastitis is present in the herd, we can easily have a nosode or oral vaccine prepared against the organism concerned. This prior determination is important in as much as there is a multiplicity of bacteria capable of causing the condition and one cannot always assume we are dealing with one of the commoner types we have mentioned. For the purpose of herd medication we usually employ the nosode in the 30th potency and have it prepared in liquid form. A 5ml vial may be added per month to the main water tank supplying the drinking water. A variation of this approach is to use certain remedies well proven in their relation to the mammary glands, e.g. Phytolacca, and Sulphur, Silicea, and Carbo Vegetabilis used in conjunction. Sub-clinical cases will obviously benefit from this approach.

In considering prevention, we must not forget the animals in the herd which are non-lactating during the summer months and consequently are at risk to Cor. Pyogenes infection – all such animals should be given a monthly dose of nosode, starting in March – heifers in calf for the first time are just as likely to succumb as older animals, and should therefore be included in the prevention programme.

(b) *Treatment of individual cases.* All outbreaks of mastitis call for the employment of various remedies according to the different symptoms, and the animal's reaction to the disease. Among the commoner remedies frequently used are the following:

1. *Belladonna 1m.* Indicated usually in the acute form postpartum. The udder shows acute swelling and redness, and pain is obvious on palpation. The animal generally may feel hot with full, bounding pulse. Dose: one every hour for four doses.
2. *Aconite 6x.* This should be employed as a routine in all acute cases, especially those which develop suddenly, possibly after exposure to cold, dry winds. It will allay tension and restlessness. Dose: one every half-hour for six doses.
3. *Apis Mellifica 6c.* This is a useful remedy for freshly calved heifers showing oedema of udder and surrounding tissues. The mammary vein is usually engorged in these cases. Dose: one every three hours for four doses.
4. *Bryonia Alba 30c.* Indicated where the udder swelling is hard and indurated. In acute cases pain will be relieved by pressure on the udder and such cases are frequently presented with the animal lying down as this appears to give relief. Chronic forms showing fibrosis should benefit from this remedy. Dose: in the acute form, one dose four-hourly for four doses. In the chronic form, one dose twice weekly for one month.

5. *Arnica Montana 30c.* When mastitis has developed as a result of injury to the udder tissue. Blood may be present in the secretion. Dose: one three times daily for three days.

6. *Bellis Perennis 6c.* Somewhat similar in its requirements to Arnica, but Bellis is probably better if the injuries are more deep than superficial, e.g. damage from teat cups which has gone on for a few days. Dose: one three times daily for four days.

7. *Phytolacca 30c.* A useful remedy both for acute and chronic cases. Acute forms may show curdled milk and clots, while in the latter, small clots may appear in mid-lactation. This is probably the most useful remedy for the average chronic case. Dose: for acute cases one three times daily for three days, followed by one daily for four days. Mastitis which appears in the form of small clots in mid-lactation will probably yield to a dose every three hours for four doses.

8. *Urtica Urens 6x.* For acute forms showing oedema which may be in the form of plaques frequently extending to the perineal area. Dose: one every hour for four doses.

9. *S.S.C. 30c.* This is a combination of Sulphur, Silicea and Carbo Veg. and has given excellent results in both acute and sub-acute cases. Clots are usually large and have a yellowish tinge, especially in the fore-milk. Dose: one three times daily for three days.

10. *Hepar Sulphuris 6x.* This low potency of Hepar will help promote suppuration and clearing of the udder contents in cases of C. Pyogenes or summer mastitis infection. Dose: one every three hours for four doses. Once the udder has been cleared of purulent material, a dose or two of a higher potency should be given to complete the cure.

11. *Silicea 200c.* Also useful in chronic cases of C. Pyogenes infection where purulent foci and sinuses have developed as a result of multiple abscesses. Dose: one twice weekly for four weeks.

Note: In acute cases remedies such as Belladonna, Bryonia and Urtica Urens may be combined as a polyvalent remedy (like S.S.C.). This will avoid the necessity for separate dosing with each remedy. The various nosodes can also be used therapeutically along with indicated remedies, a dose a day for three consecutive days being sufficient.

12. *Ipecac 30c.* This is a useful remedy for controlling intra-mammary bleeding which results in 'pink milk', or even more frank bleeding. Dose: one three times daily for three days.

13. Heat Prostration

There are two types of heat attack which may affect cattle: (A) sunstroke and (B) heat exhaustion. The former is the name given to the syndrome produced by direct rays of the sun on animals (especially dairy or fine-skinned subjects) while the latter signifies that state of prostration due to an accumulation of body heat.

A. Sunstroke. Direct rays of the sun on the head may produce dilation of cerebral blood-vessels which in severe cases can cause paralysis.

SYMPTOMS. Excitement and restlessness are quickly evident and in the less acute case paralysis of certain muscles takes place, finally leading to failure of the respiratory centre.

TREATMENT.
1. *Aconitum Napellus 12x.* This remedy given at once will help calm the animal and reduce excitement. Dose: one every half-hour for four doses.
2. *Belladonna 1m.* A most useful remedy for cerebral congestion. Generally there may be visible throbbing of surface vessels, with excitement and dilated pupils. Dose: one every half-hour for four doses. It should be alternated with Aconitum.
3. *Glonoine 30c.* One of the main remedies for exposure to sun. The animal exhibits signs of pain in the head, such as throwing the head against any convenient object or banging on the ground. Recumbency is usual with unsteadiness of movement if made to rise. This remedy will do much to reduce the tension in the cerebral blood vessels. Dose: one every hour for four doses.

B. Heat exhaustion. Accumulation of body heat may arise after exposure to a long spell of hot weather when the heat builds up in the body. It can be made worse by exercise. Factors which may influence this condition apart from heat are lack of proper oxygenation, fatigue, and insufficient intake of water, together with unnecessary handling, during prolonged hot weather.

SYMPTOMS.   Rapid respirations are a constant sign along with depression and anorexia. The mouth is usually open and frothy mucus accumulates. A rapid pulse is present, while an extremely high temperature is constant. The conjunctivae become congested and motor reflexes are lost.

TREATMENT.
1. *Glonoine 30c.*   As Glonoine 30c for Sunstroke.
2. *Natrum Muriaticum 30c.*   A useful remedy for stabilising the salt metabolism and preventing loss. Dose: one every three hours for four doses.
3. *Sulphur 30c.*   This remedy is useful for reducing the effects of heat generally, enabling the animal to make a quicker recovery. Dose: one dose every two hours for four doses.

The administration of these remedies will help the action of cold water applications, which are always extremely valuable in reducing heat.

14. Bacterial Diseases

1. Leptospirosis. This disease may affect one or a group of animals with variable symptoms in each animal.

ETIOLOGY. There are two main species of leptospira concerned: (1) *L. Pomona* and *L. Icterohaemorrhagica*. The latter affects mainly calves and younger animals and has been dealt with in the disease of calves section. Infection by L. Pomona may be spread by contact with carrier pigs which excrete the organism in the urine.

CLINICAL SIGNS. There is an incubation period of about two days after which fever sets in with a rise in temperature to 106°F or 107°F. Severe and mild forms of the disease are recognised. In the severe form the onset is sudden and comes after a short period of inappetance and reduced milk yield. Signs of liver involvement appear with jaundice of visible mucous membranes. Milk becomes bloodstained and assumes an orange or brown colour. Blood-pigment appears in the urine, giving it a port-wine appearance. Abortions are fairly constant. Milder forms show similar but less pronounced symptoms lasting only a few days. The udder becomes spongy and soft, and rarely assumes its firm character. Haemoglobinuria is present as well as jaundice.

TREATMENT. The following remedies are worthy of consideration:
1. *Aconitum Napellus 12x.* Should be given as early as possible. Dose: one every half-hour for four doses.
2. *Crotalus Horridus 200c.* A very good remedy for controlling liver complications and reducing haemorrhages and jaundice. Dose: one every half-hour for four doses.
3. *Berberis Vulgaris 30c.* Suitable for the milder case. Will control liver dysfunction and reduce haemoglobinuria. Dose: one three times daily for two days.
4. *Phosphorus 1m.* Another valuable liver remedy. Will also control the tendency to haemorrhages. Faeces are generally clay-coloured. Dose: one daily for one week.

5. *Ipecacuanha 30c.* A good anti-haemorrhagic remedy and will be found useful especially for controlling the excretion of blood in the milk. Dose: one three times daily for three days.

2. Tetanus. This is an infectious disease resulting from the absorption of specific toxin and its subsequent fixation to the central nervous system.

ETIOLOGY. The cause is a bacterium – *Clostridium tetani* – an organism which can produce its toxin only in the absence of free oxygen. Hence the danger of tetanus arising as a result of deep punctured wounds or of those deprived of free oxygen. Occasionally tetanus is described as idiopathic, when it arises in the absence of a visible source or wound.

CLINICAL SIGNS. After an incubation period which may be up to three weeks, muscle spasm may be seen along with a stiffness of movement. Respirations are increased and the patient may show difficulty in chewing or swallowing. As the disease progresses the muscle rigidity and spasms become more intense and this coincides with an anxious expression and extended head. The alae nasi are dilated to allow for the maximum intake of air. There is increased awareness of external stimuli. Abdominal bloat is a fairly constant sign in the later stages as also is trismus.

TREATMENT. If the disease is suspected or thought likely to develop as a result of a typical wound, besides the routine administration of antitoxin the following two remedies should be given in alternation, one every hour for five doses each.
1. *Hypericum 1m.* This is the main remedy for wounds where damage to nerve endings has taken place.
2. *Ledum Palustre 6c.* Useful particularly where the wound is of a deep punctured type. Tissue surrounding the wound becomes cold and bluish.
If the disease has advanced these two remedies will still be useful but in addition the following remedies should be considered.
3. *Strychninum 200c.* For muscular rigidity and the tendency for limbs to be extended along with arched back. Dose: one three times daily for five days.

4. *Cuprum Metallicum 1m.* For the early stages of muscular cramp and spasm. The underlying skin becomes bluish. Dose: one twice daily for four days.
5. *Nux Vomica 1m.* This remedy may be useful in controlling digestive symptoms and helping prevent the onset of bloat. Dose: one twice daily for five days.
6. *Colchicum 200c.* If bloat develops to a marked degree, this remedy may bring relief, used in conjunction with other indicated remedies. Dose: one every half-hour for five doses.

3. Botulism. This particular poisoning is sometimes met with in cattle grazing on phosphorus-deficient pastures in certain countries where range conditions obtain. It is assumed that the poison is ingested when the animal eats bones in an endeavour to satisfy a need for phosphorus.

ETIOLOGY. The toxin is secreted by an organism named *Clostridium botulinum*. This may also secrete the poison in decaying animal or vegetable material, which could be consumed by cattle in periods of drought, or in the absence of more suitable fodder.

CLINICAL SIGNS. The toxin attacks peripheral nerves and may lead to a variety of symptoms. There is an absence of fever while paralysis is seen in the muscles affecting swallowing and mastication, and also in those of the limbs. Animals walk with difficulty, and when made to do so, assume a stiff gait with the head carried near the ground. There is usually excessive salivation due to paralysis of the nerves of deglutition, which also causes the tongue to be protruded.

TREATMENT. In cases not too far advanced, the following remedies will be of value:
1. *Gelsemium 200c.* Where paralytic signs are seen principally in the throat causing difficulty in swallowing. Dose: one every hour for five doses.
2. *Lathyrus Sativa 1m.* This remedy will also benefit peripheral paralysis of throat and mouth, with, in addition, a beneficial effect on the nerves governing locomotion, especially in the upper forelimb. Dose: one every hour for four doses, followed by one per day for four days.

3. *Curare 30c.* For milder cases showing muscular stiffness with difficulty in walking properly, particularly seen in the front legs. Dose: one three times daily for five days.
4. *Conium Maculatum 200c.* A suitable remedy when paralytic symptoms are seen mainly in the hind-limbs. The animal is sometimes unable to rise. Dose: one twice daily for one week.
5. *Plumbum. Metallicum 30c.* This is also a good remedy for general paralysis of limb muscles, especially the fore limbs. Paralysis may be preceded by loss of sensation in the affected part. Dose: one twice daily for one week.

4. Actinomycosis and Actinobacillosis. These two conditions, although caused by different bacteria, are usually classed together. They cause granulomatous swellings on the jaw and the soft tissues of the tongue and palate, with occasional spread to the stomachs.

ETIOLOGY. Actinomycosis is caused by a bacterium known as Actinomyces bovis and Actinobacillosis by Actinobacillus lignieresi, often in association with pyogenic bacteria. Invasion of the tissues usually takes place through small wounds in the mouth.

SYMPTOMS. Actinomycosis appears as a swelling of bone first noticeable especially on the mandible, where the majority of the lesions of this disease occur. This swelling may be slow-growing or it may develop rapidly. Actinobacillosis of the tongue is usually referred to as 'wooden' or 'timber tongue', and causes the tongue to become thick and hard. Salivation is profuse but not frothy, and in severe cases the tongue may become ulcerated. If the throat glands are affected, swelling of the region is obvious while involvement of the rumen or reticulum causes bloat and impairment of digestion.

TREATMENT.
A. Actinomycosis
1. *Hekla Lava 1m.* This is a most useful remedy for bony swellings especially of the head bones. Dose: one daily for ten days. It may be necessary to continue treatment over a longer period with lower potencies.
2. *Kali Hydriodicum 200c.* This remedy has a specific action on the infection and used to be used allopathically by injection. It gives much better results when used in potency. Dose: one twice daily for ten days.

3. *Acidum Fluoricum 30c.* The action of this remedy is somewhat similar to that of Hekla Lava, but is more suitable for those cases showing ulceration of overlying skin and caries of bone with discharge. Dose: one twice daily for two weeks.

B. Actinobacillosis.
1. *Kali Hydriodicum 200c.* As for Actinomycosis above.
2. *Mercurius Iodatus Flavus 30c.* A useful remedy for swollen throat glands, especially those on the right side. Dose: one three times daily for five days.
3. *Mercurius Iodatus Ruber 30c.* This is also a useful remedy for swollen throat glands, but acts better on the left side of the neck. Dose: as above, Merc. Iod. Fl. This remedy should also be useful for cases involving the tongue, especially when the posterior part is affected.

15. Virus Diseases

1. Cow Pox. This is a vesicular and pustular disease characterised by eruptions on the skin.

ETIOLOGY. A filterable virus is the cause which is easily transmitted from animal to animal.

CLINICAL SIGNS. The incubation period is from 4–7 days. There may be an early transient fever, but this may go unnoticed. The udder and teats show sensitivity to touch in the early stages. The lesions are usually confined to the teats and skin of the udder, and progress through the recognised stages of papule, vesicle, pustule and scab formation. The papular stage lasts about two days and the following vesicular stage appears about the third or fourth day. The vesicles contain a straw-coloured fluid. This becomes pustular about the eighth day and is followed by the scab or healing stage.

TREATMENT.
Although this disease is invariably mild, the use of one or other of the following remedies will cut short the infective process, and prevent secondary infection of pustules which frequently occurs if the condition is allowed to run its course.
1. *Antimonium Crudum 6c.* This remedy is associated with typical papular and pustular skin lesions, especially with a generally dry skin. Signs of indigestion may be present. Dose: one three times daily for three days.
2. *Cuprum Aceticum 6c.* A leading remedy for pox-like eruptions frequently accompanied by cramps and spasms of groups of muscles. Diarrhoea may also be present. Dose: one three times daily for three days.
3. *Kali Bichromicum 30c.* The pustules assume a crater-like discrete form with yellowish base and discharge. Dose: one twice daily for five days.
4. *Variolinum 30c or Vaccinium 200c.* Either of these nosodes will be found of value either by themselves or used in conjunc-

tion with one or the other of the above remedies. Dose: one daily for three days.

5. *Ranunculus Bulbosus 6c.* Another useful remedy for the vesicular stage especially if more prominent on the udder. Dose: one three times daily for five days.

PREVENTION. A course of Variolinum 30c will be found of benefit in controlling the disease on a herd basis. One dose should be given to all cows and repeated at monthly intervals for three months.

2. Malignant Catarrhal Fever. This disease affects cattle of all ages, more commonly in 2-year-olds and upwards. It is acutely infectious. Various mucous membranes are affected by acute inflammation particularly the respiratory, but changes also occur in the central nervous and digestive systems.

ETIOLOGY. Believed to be caused by a virus, possibly gaining entrance to the system via the mucous membrane of the respiratory or digestive tract.

SYMPTOMS. Early signs appear suddenly and are characterised by very high temperature, staring coat and watery ocular discharge. Congestion of respiratory mucous membranes leads to dyspnoea and a rapid increase in breathing. Pulse rate is increased while colour changes affect the muzzle which becomes deep red. Nasal discharge of reddish brown mucus occurs. As the disease progresses, digestive changes occur evidenced by diarrhoea and tenesmus. Affection of the central nervous system results in hypersensitivity of the skin and sometimes in convulsions and mania. The redness of the muzzle is superseded by a scabby fibrinous deposit which peels easily, leaving a necrotic surface. The nasal discharge at this stage becomes thick and purulent. The cornea of the eye begins to show opacity which later becomes dense with occasionally ulceration. The necrosis of the nuzzle extends to the dental pad, leaving raw haemorrhagic areas. Muscular twitchings and dehydration are constant accompaninents in the later stages.

TREATMENT.

1. *Aconitum 30c.* Should be given as early as possible in the febrile stage. One dose every half-hour for four doses.

2. *Ferrum Phosph 12x.*   This should follow Aconitum, giving one dose every hour for three doses.
3. *Arsenicum Album 1m.*   Will help control the acrid lachry-mation and dehydration – the early picture of the disease strongly suggests this remedy. One dose four times in one day, three hours apart.
4. *Antimonium Tartaricum 30c.*   Should influence the respiratory symptoms and help reduce the bronchial inflammation and accompanying mucus. One dose three times daily for one week.
5. *Kreosotum 200c.*   For the changes occuring on the muzzle and dental pad, this remedy will be of use, giving one dose three times daily for three days.
6. *Acidum Nitricum 200c.*   Ulceration around the mouth and on the tongue should be helped by Nitric Acid. It may also have a beneficial effect on corneal ulceration and the severe diarrhoea. The latter probably being due to ulceration of the intestinal mucous membranes. One dose should be given thrice daily for four days.
7. *Silicea 200c.*   When opacity of the cornea occurs. The early ad-ministration of Silicea should help prevent further opacity deve-loping. This remedy may have to be repeated at less frequent intervals depending on the initial response. Dose: one twice weekly for one month.
8. *Strychninum 30c.*   Has been found of use in controlling muscu-lar twitchings which may develop in the later stages. One dose night and morning for ten days may be needed.
9. *Pyrogen 1m.*   If symptoms develop which bring about a weak thready pulse accompanying the very high temperature, Pyrogen will give rapid relief. It is less likely to help if the pulse remains full and rapid. Dose: one every three hours for four doses.

3.   Vesicular Stomatitis.   This is a febrile disease characterised by the development of vesicles on various parts of the body.

ETIOLOGY.   A specific virus is responsible.

SYMPTOMS.   There may be a short incubation period of up to 36 hours in adult animals, but is much longer in young animals. There is an initial pyrexia with accompanying depression. Salivation is prominent. The temperature rise corresponds to the development of the vesicles which on rupturing bring about a reduction in temperature. Saliva at first fluid soon becomes sticky and thick and accompanies a smacking sound. Mucous nasal discharge may be present. Vesicles develop on gums inside the lips and on the muzzle. There may be coalescence of groups of vesicles, giving rise to a large ulcerated surface when they rupture. Vesicles may develop on teats and udder where the healing process is usually much slower than on the mouth. The feet are sometimes involved, vesicles arising along the coronary band and in the inter-digital space.

TREATMENT.
1. *Aconitum 30c.* Should precede other treatment if possible when signs of inappetance show and the febrile stage is being ushered in. Give one dose every half-hour for four doses.
2. *Borax 6c.* Almost specific once vesicles have developed in the mouth accompanying salivation. It will promote rapid healing even after the vesicles have ruptured. Give one dose thrice daily for one week.
3. *Ranunculus Bulbosus 6c.* This is a useful remedy for the treatment of vesicles on body parts distinct from the oral region, e.g. on teats and udder. Give one dose thrice daily for five days.
4. *Antimonium Crudum 6c.* This remedy is more suitable for the treatment on rough-coated, thick-skinned animals with a tendency to develop horny callosities. It will also help control the nasal discharges accompanying the disease. The healing ulcers assume a yellowish colour. Dose: one thrice daily for ten days.
5. *Cuprum Aceticum 6c.* Skin lesions may be accompanied by muscular involvement, such as stiffness and trembling. Miliary rashes accompany the vesicles. Dose: one twice daily for two weeks.
6. *Natrum Muriaticum 30c.* A remedy which will aid the healing process of foot lesions as well as favouring the healing process in the mouth. Thirst may be prominent when the remedy is indicated. Dose: one thrice daily for one week.
7. *Variolinum 30c.* The smallpox nosode can be used both therapeutically and in prevention. One dose per day for three consecutive days may be given concurrently with other remedies. For preventive purposes it may limit development of the disease if given in two doses, one week apart to susceptible animals. This however is less effective than the specific nosode which may be prepared from vesicular contents.

4. Ephemeral Fever. This disease is characterised by inflammatory changes in the musculo-skeletal system and associated lymphatic glands. It is vector borne.

ETIOLOGY.   The virus is associated with the leucocyte fraction of the blood and is transmitted mainly by the sandfly. The disease is commonest in adult cattle.

SYMPTOMS.   The disease usually runs an acute course but is rarely fatal in properly treated cattle. Following a rise in temperature up to 106°F, inappetance and variable digestive symptoms appear, e.g. there may be looseness of bowel movement or constipation. Respiration and heart are both increased while milk yield falls. Nasal and eye discharges occur. Muscular involvement sets in, evidenced by shivering, weakness and stiffness which eventually leads to recumbency in many cases, but frequently the animal retains a normal stance.

TREATMENT.   The main remedies to be considered are:
1. *Aconitum 12x.*   For the initial period of fever; one dose every half-hour for four doses.
2. *Arsenicum Album 1m.*   Should be used to control ocular and nasal discharges. It may also help restore normal respiration and bowel movement. Dose: one three times daily for three days.
3. *Bryonia 30c.*   When involvement of pleura and pericardium occur leading to increased respiration and heart rate, this remedy will be found useful. Dose: one every three hours for four doses.
4. *Nux Vomica 1m.*   Digestive disorders associated with lack of rumenation and anorexia will benefit. Should also restore normal motion. Dose: one per day for seven days.
5. *Strychnine 6c.*   Will help control muscular twitching and shivering. Dose: one three times daily for three days.
6. *Cuprum Metallicum 1m.*   For muscular crampings and clonic muscle movements. Dose: one per day for five days.
7. *Carcinosin 200c.*   This nosode will be found useful for involvement of lymphatic glands frequently bringing about resolution in inflammation. Dose: one dose twice weekly for two weeks.

5.   Bovine Malignant Catarrh.   Characteristic of this disease is a catarrhal inflammation of the upper respiratory epithelium, together with similar changes in the alimentary canal. The central nervous system and lymphatic system are also involved.

ETIOLOGY. The disease is caused by a herpes virus which may be spread by insect vectors or by direct contact.

SYMPTOMS. There is a fairly long incubation period of 3–8 weeks which is followed by a rise in temperature – up to 107°F – loss of milk yield, depression and loss of appetite. Discharges of muco-purulent material occur from nose and eyes. Respiratory distress is evident. There may be oedematous infiltration of eyelids. Necrotic patches soon appear inside the mouth, especially on the gums and corners of lips. This necrosis extends also to the muzzle which eventually become scabby, and also to the teats, udder and feet. When the virus invades the central nervous system, inco-ordination, paralysis and convulsions may appear. Lymphatic glands are invariably swollen. In the alimentary sphere there may be dysentery, while involvement of the kidney leads to the presence of blood in the urine. Corneal opacity is a fairly constant sign, in varying degrees.

TREATMENT. Milder forms of the disease will be helped towards recovery by the following remedies, according to the preponderance of symptoms displayed.
1. *Aconitum 12x.* For the early febrile stage, if given as soon as possible. Dose: one every half-hour for four doses.
2. *Arsenicum Album 1m.* Will influence the ocular and nasal discharges especially in the early non-purulent stage. Diarrhoea and dysentery should also be helped. Dose: one every two hours for four doses.
3. *Acidum Nitricum 200c.* This is an important remedy for controlling epithelial ulceration, especially in the mouth, around the lips and muzzle. If given early it should help prevent subsequent necrosis. Dose: one three times daily for five days.
4. *Phosphorus 1m.* This remedy is useful for involvement of the respiratory tract where inflammation may extend to lung tissue. It will also act on liver and kidneys, preventing threatened fatty degeneration and nephritis. Dose: one four times daily three hours apart, followed by one daily for one week.
5. *Silicea 200c.* Should favourably influence corneal opacity, helping to reduce and absorb scarring. Dose: one daily for seven days.

6. *Plumbum 1m.* If involvement of the central nervous system leads to single limb weakness. Dose: one daily for one week.

7. *Lathyrus Sativus 1m.* Will be of use in cases showing peripheral paralysis and inco-ordination, with muscle trembling. Dose: one twice daily for fourteen days.

8. *Belladonna 1m or 200c.* Convulsions should respond to the use of this remedy given in half-hour doses for four hours.

9. *Rhus Toxicodendron 1m.* Redness and inflammation of mouth and throat before the onset of necrosed areas should be helped. Gastritis will also benefit. Dose: one three times daily for four days.

10. *Mercurius Corrosivus 200c.* If lesions are accompanied by purulent discharges and slimy dysentery this remedy should help; also if purulent conjuctivitis sets in. Dose: one three times daily for one week.

11. *Carcinosin 200c.* When one of the main signs is acute involvement of lymphatic glands. Dose: one daily for four days.

6. Infectious Bovine Rhinotracheitis. This viral disease is associated with upper respiratory and ocular discharges and runs a relatively short course. Abortions are also common.

ETIOLOGY. A herpes virus is the cause which is common in animals under six months of age, and is spread by droplet infection and direct contact.

SYMPTOMS. There is a variable incubation period of 3–20 days, followed by high temperature and loss of appetite. The nasal mucous membrane becomes inflamed and discharges occur from the eyes. Increased salivation is a prominent feature. Secondary pneumonia may set in if the disease is allowed to proceed unchecked. Conjunctivitis is a fairly common lesion, the eyelids becoming thickened and rough. Abortions commonly occur in prolonged infections. Brain involvement has been recorded leading to convulsions.

TREATMENT.

1. *Aconitum 12x.* Should be given at half-hourly intervals for four doses as soon as febrile symptoms are evident.

2. *Arsenicum Album 1m.* This remedy may cut short the development of the disease if given when nasal and ocular discharges are first noticed and before they become purulent. Dose: one every hour for four doses.

3. *Mercurius Corrosivus 200c.* When salivation is prominent and discharges become purulent. Dose: one three times daily for three days.

4. *Drosera 9c.* Should control inflammation of larynx and trachea and help the associated cough which is not always present. Dose: one three times daily for four days.

5. *Arsenicum Iodatum 30c.* Will also aid the inflammation in the respiratory tract, especially deeper or lower involvement than the trachea. Dose: one twice daily for one week.

6. *Antimonium Tartaricum 30c.* When secondary bronchopneumonia occurs with muco-purulent sputum and rattling bronchial sounds. Dose: one three times daily for five days.

7. *Kali Bichromatum 200c.* If nasal discharges become thick and chronic leading to tough, stringy, yellow nasal plugs. Dose: one twice daily for one week.

8. *Argentum Nitricum 30c.* A useful remedy for controlling conjunctivitis. Dose: one three times daily for five days.

9. *Euphrasia.* A lotion made up of 1/10 will be found useful for bathing the eyes, used in conjunction with the above remedy.

10. *Belladonna 1m.* If convulsions threaten, an hourly dose of this remedy for four hours will help. There will probably be an accompanying hot skin and full bounding pulse.

7. Papillomatosis. This is the name given to the common wart formation of cattle frequently encountered in the younger animal.

ETIOLOGY. A virus which is host specific.

SYMPTOMS. An incubation period of a little more than two months occurs in natural infection. The warts may be attached to the skin by a neck or pedicle (pedunculated warts) or flattened on the skin (sessile warts). They may appear on any surface but are most commonly seen on the head, around the eyes and on the shoulder region. They appear as a dry roughened mass resembling the surface of a cauliflower. In the cow, teat involvement is common. Frequently the warts have a pinkish tinge and the pedunculated variety tend to bleed easily.

TREATMENT. The effects of homoeopathic treatment take some time to appear and it may be two or three months after cessation of medication before results are seen. The main remedies to be considered are:

1. *Thuja 30c or 200c.* The most important remedy when dealing with pedunculated warts possessing a foul smell and which bleed easily. Dose: one daily for fourteen days.
2. *Causticum 6c.* This remedy may influence the sessile wart whether singly or in clusters. Dose: one twice daily for two weeks.
3. *Calcarea Carbonica 30c.* A useful remedy for the small flat warts which develop on the teats of heifers and cows. Dose: one twice weekly for one month.
4. *Dulcamara 200c.* For large flat smooth warts which develop mainly on the head and limbs. Dose: one daily for seven days.
5. *Acidum Nitricum 200c.* Warts are large and sharp-edged They tend to bleed easily. Dose: one daily for seven days.
6. *Sabina 6c.* A little-used but sometimes effective remedy. Warts are more usually seen in genital areas. Dose: twice daily for fourteen days.

8. Bovine Ulcerative Mammilitis. This disease is characterised by skin ulceration of teats and udder in milking cows. Younger animals are more prone to infection.

ETIOLOGY. A herpes virus which produces disease mainly in autumn and early winter.

SYMPTOMS. A period of up to 12 days is necessary for the development of lesions, which do not appear anywhere but on teats and udder. Depending on the length of time the cow has calved, lesions develop on teats (later calving) or on the udder (recent calving). If there is severe udder oedema in the freshly calved animal, the lesions tend to be more pronounced. Vesicles first appear at the base of the teat which coalesce and rupture, leaving a large raw surface. In very severe outbreaks the teat swells, assumes a bluish colour and exudes serum. Less pronounced lesions comprise shallow ulcers following papule formation.

TREATMENT.

1. *Kali Bichromicum 200c.* For shallow ulcers with yellowish tenacious exudation. Margins of ulcers are sharply defined. Dose: one twice daily for one week.
2. *Antimonium Crudum 6c.* Useful in the early stages if the skin on teats or udder remains dry. Dose: one thrice daily for five days.
3. *Acidum Muriaticum 6c.* For ulcers which quickly become foulsmelling and assume a livid appearance. Dose: one three times daily for four days.
4. *Mercurius Solubilis 30c.* For those cases where the skin remains moist because of serum exudation. Ulcers are irregular in outline and show a pimply rash surrounding them. There is a tendency to local suppuration with yellow crusty scabs. Dose: one three times daily for four days.
5. *Arsenicum Album 1m.* For dry skin showing oedema. Ulcers are dark red and may discharge dark offensive material. There is a tendency to gangrene. Dose: one daily for one week.
6. *Carbo Vegetabilis 200c.* When this remedy is indicated there is usually bluish discolouration and is therefore useful in the more severe or acute outbreak. There may be peripheral bleeding around the ulcer margins. Dose: one twice daily for four days.

9. Louping Ill. This disease takes the form of an encephalomyelitis associated with tick-infested pastures in certain parts of the country.

ETIOLOGY. A neurotropic virus is responsible and the organism gains entrance to the system through the bite of an infected vector – the tick *Ixodes ricinus*. There is a seasonal incidence of tick activity, viz. spring and autumn and the disease is most commonly encountered at these times.

SYMPTOMS. If susceptible animals are put to infested grazings they soon show signs of disturbance of the central nervous system, e.g. muscle tremors, exaggerated movements, excitability and an increased response to external stimuli. The feet may be carried in an unduly high action. There may be knuckling at the fetlocks followed by recumbency. Frequently the disease takes a mild form.

TREATMENT. According to the symptoms exhibited by any one animal, the following remedies may be indicated:

1. *Aconitum Napellus 12x.* Should be given in the early stages of fever if possible, when the disease is first suspected. Dose: one every half-hour for four doses.
2. *Agaricus Muscarius 30c.* For those cases where the patient shows a tendency to fall backwards. There is much twitching of head muscles and excitability, together with exaggerated high stepping. Dose: one three times daily for one week.
3. *Cicuta Virosa 200c.* When this remedy is indicated there is frequently deviation of the head to one side, with contraction of neck muscles. The gait is unsteady and muscular spasms occur. Dose: one twice daily for five days.
4. *Curare 30c.* For incoordination of gait with a tendency to knuckling and general muscular weakness, especially in the forelimbs. Dose: one twice daily for two weeks.
5. *Conium Maculatum 30c.* Indicated when muscular weakness or partial paralysis begins in the hind limbs and tends to move forward. The animal rises with difficulty and stumbles frequently. Dose: one twice daily for one week.

PREVENTION. An effective oral vaccine (nosode) exists and animals at risk should be given two doses one month apart, the second dose being timed fourteen days before the animals are put on to infested grazing. An inter-current dose of Sulphur 30c reinforces the immunity.

16. Affections of the Female Reproductive Tract

1. Coital Vesicular Exanthema. Vesicular Vaginitis. This disease is characterised by the formation of vesicles on the mucous membranes of the vulva and vagina. Bulls are also affected.

ETIOLOGY. A virus has been identified as the cause and infection is spread by coitus.

SYMPTOMS. The animal exhibits straining and restlessness. Urination is frequent and there may be stamping of the feet and switching of the tail. A whitish vaginal discharge is present, soiling the tail and vulval region. Small vesicles cover the vaginal mucous membrane, while swelling of the vulva occurs. The vesicles tend to coalesce with a serous exudate. Secondary infection of these lesions results in a purulent discharge. The bull shows similar lesions on the penis and prepuce. Abortions do not occur.

TREATMENT.
1. *Cantharis 30c.* Frequent urination with straining and vesicular inflammation of the genital tract call for this remedy. Dose: one three times daily for five days.
2. *Hydrastis 30c.* Thick catarrhal exudate is an indication for this remedy. Dose: one twice daily for one week.
3. *Mercuris Corrosivus 200c.* For severe inflammation with secondary infection of ulcerated surfaces. Dose: one three times daily for three days.
4. *Acidum Nitricum 200c.* A very useful remedy for the treatment of ulcerated surfaces of the body orifices, with watery discharge. Dose: one daily for one week.
5. *Rhus Toxicodendron.* A remedy which is indicated in the early vesicular stage. The surrounding mucous membrane is dark red. Dose: one daily for five days.
The vaginal mucous membrane should be irrigated with a solu-

tion of Calendula in a strength of 1/10. The penis and prepuce of the bull should be similarly treated.

2.   Granular Vaginitis.   Sometimes referred to as Nodular Vaginitis, this condition is associated with the presence of lymphoid nodules on the vulva and posterior vagina. Bulls may develop the nodules on the penis and prepuce.

ETIOLOGY.   The actual cause has not been determined but is possibly of an infectious nature.

SYMPTOMS.   Heifers are more severly affected than the older animals. The typical nodule of lymphoid tissue appears on the posterior vagina and may be under the epithelium or protrude above it. Severe cases show a reddening of the surrounding mucous membrane which assumes a granular appearance. Secondary infection may lead to a purulent exudate. In the bull the penis and prepuce are similarly affected.

TREATMENT.   As for Vesicular Vaginitis. In addition the following remedies will be of use.
1. *Calcarea Fluorica 30c.* A very good tissue remedy which should have a softening effect on the lymphoid nodules, hastening their disappearance. Dose: one twice weekly for one month.
2. *Thuja Occidentalis 6c.* Also indicated where tumours and nodules develop. Dose: one twice daily for two weeks.

3.   Vibriosis.   This infectious disease of the genital tract of cattle is characterised by infertility and abortion.

ETIOLOGY.   The causal organism is a bacterium – *Vibrio fetus* – and infection is transmitted through coitus.

MAIN CHARACTERISTICS OF THE DISEASE.   There may be an abnormally long oestrus cycle, a period of up to eight weeks being possible. This is due to death and resorption or abortion of foetus, the abortion being undetected. The age group most susceptible is two to three years. Older animals develop an immunity and therefore show less involvement. Abortions are commonest around the fifth or sixth month, the placenta being expelled with the foetus in the majority of cases. Only the genital organs of the female are affected, the disease causing changes in the placenta of the pregnant animal resulting in separation and expulsion, preceded by a blood-tinged mucous discharge.

TREATMENT.   This should be directed towards the cervicitis which occurs after abortion and expulsion of the placenta. The following remedies have been found helpful.

1. *Calcarea Phosphorica 30c.*   The mucus is thin, clear, and blood-stained. Dose: one three times daily for two days followed by one every second day for three doses.

2. *Hydrastis 30c.*   Indicated when the catarrhal discharge is muco-purulent due to secondary infection. Dose: one twice daily for one week.

3. *Sabina 6c.*   A useful remedy for controlling past-partum blood-stained discharges sometimes containing whole bright red blood. Dose: one three times daily for three days.

4. *Secale 30c.*   Discharges of blood also indicate this remedy, the difference here being that the blood is dark. Dose: one twice daily for one week.

PREVENTION.   A nosode made from infective vaginal mucus may be used to protect young stock. One dose of 30c potency should be given every three months from one year until the animal is put to the bull. Thereafter in-calf animals should receive one dose per month.

4.   Trichomoniasis.   This genital disease is associated with abortion and consequent sterility. Heifers are more susceptible than older animals. Infection rarely extends beyond the genital tract.

ETIOLOGY.   The protozoon parasite *T. fetus* is commonly accepted as the cause.

SYMPTOMS.   The disease is spread by coitus and frequently the only signs are irregularities in the oestrus cycle, e.g. failure of conception on the part of a number of animals or abortion occuring between three and five months. The presence of pus in the uterus is a fairly constant feature. The foetus is usually expelled with the placenta, but occasionally retention of a dead foetus leads to a muco-purulent discharge once pyometritis develops. Sometimes the uterine seal remains intact leading to a build-up of purulent material of a non-toxic nature.

TREATMENT.
1. *Hydrastis 30c.* This is a very good remedy for any catarrhal condition arising as a result of inflammation affecting mucous membranes. It is therefore applicable to uterine conditions discharging muco-purulent material. Dose: one three times daily for four days.
2. *Caulophyllum 30c.* A remedy which also aids expulsion of uterine fluids. It has a specific action on the uterus and is therefore indicated in those cases where the uterine seal remains intact. Under its influence the seal will relax allowing discharge of uterine contents. Dose: one three-hourly for four doses.
3. *Sepia 200c.* Sepia has a beneficial action on the entire female genital system and will aid materially in regulating the oestrus cycle. Dose: one twice weekly for one month.
4. *Apis 30c.* If suspected in the early stages apis will help control the oedema which affects the lining of the uterus and thus limit extension of the pathological process. Dose: one three times daily for three days.

The use of a nosode made from a culture of *T. fetus* will be helpful in controlling the disease on a herd basis. Susceptible animals should receive one dose per month for three months before service, using a 30c potency.

5. Puerperal Metritis. This condition is an inflammation of the uterus associated with parturition, resulting in systemic involvement which can lead to severe illness.

ETIOLOGY. During the puerperium the lining of the uterus is commonly the seat of bacterial multiplication. Any condition which delays the course of uterine involution tends to favour such infection, e.g. dystocia or retained placenta.

SYMPTOMS. An initial rise of temperature is followed by lack of appetite and general malaise. Respirations are increased and recumbency is usual. The pulse is either weak and thready or full and tense, and the expression is anxious. Acute metritis generally leads to involvement of the peritoneum, the inflammatory process being felt as a board-like mass on palpatation of the sub-lumbar fossa. The vagina and vulva may be inflamed and dark red. Discharge is not always present, but if present it usually contains dark blood.

TREATMENT.
1. *Aconitum Napellus 6c.*   The earlier this remedy is given, the more likely it is that a successful outcome will ensue. It is particularly indicated in those cases which arise with sudden intensity. Its action helps allay shock and reduce fears. Dose: one every half-hour for six doses.
2. *Belladonna 1m.*   A useful remedy when there is a full, bounding pulse, hot skin and dilated pupils, with signs of impending delirium. Dose: one every hour for five doses.
3. *Echinacea 3x.*   Indicated where systemic involvement is rapid and signs of septicaemia are present. Temperature remains high, and respirations are shallow. This is a remedy which acts best in lower potencies. Dose: one every two hours for four doses.
4. *Sabina 6c.*   This is a useful remedy when the trouble is associated with retention of placenta. Discharges are blood-stained or may be of pure blood, which is usually bright red. Dose: one every two hours for four doses.
5. *Secale 30c.*   This has a somewhat similar picture to Sabina, but discharges contain dark fluid blood, and the animal has a lean or cadaverous appearance. Signs of disturbance to the peripheral circulation may be present, e.g. cold extremities and lack of sensation. Dose: one three times daily for four days.
6. *Lachesis.*   If the condition manifests itself in a haemorrhagic form with bluish discolouration of visible parts and swelling of limbs, this remedy may prove useful. Frequently the throat is swollen leading to difficulty in swallowing. Dose: one three times daily for four doses.

17. Infertility in the Cow and Irregularities of the Oestrus Cycle

Infertility may have its origins in ovarian dysfunction or in abnormalities of the uterus and fallopian tubes, and may be temporary or permanent. In the absence of pregnancy oestrus occurs all the year round, the cycle appearing every 19–21 days and showing again about 48–56 days after parturition. The oestrus period lasts 12 hours in winter and about 48 hours in summer. A prolonged cycle frequently denotes late ovulation and could be a reason for delayed conception. A short cycle might mean early ovulation but would not interfere with fertilisation.

Five stages are recognised in the oestrus cycle, viz:

1. Pro-oestrus. This is the period of preparation in which the Graafian follicle is growing and leads to accumulation of follicular fluid. This fluid contains a steroid hormone – oestradiol – which along with other substances known as oestrol and oestriol constitutes oestrogen.

2. Oestrus. This is the period of excitement or desire in which the ovary has matured along with the Graafian follicle.

3. Metoestrus. The day after oestrus usually leads to rupture of the follicle and expulsion of the ovum. The follicular cavity is filled by the embryonic corpus luteum. This body secretes progesterone, the function of which is to prepare the endometrum for implantation of the fertilised ovum. At the same time oestrogen is inhibited and maturation of other follicles suppressed. It also controls mammary gland development.

4. Dioestrus. During this period the uterine walls thicken and the uterine glands are active. Firmness of the corpus luteum is the rule. If pregnancy supervenes this condition persists, but in the absence of pregnancy the corpus luteum is resorbed, the withdrawal of progesterone initiating a new oestrus cycle.

5. Anoestrus. This is a period of inactivity which may occur as a sequel to dioestrus or instead of it. It normally persists for a period of about seven or eight weeks after parturition.

Let us now review the main causes of infertility where we might reasonably expect homoeopathic medication to be of benefit. These may be summarised as follows:

(a) Temperamental factors, (b) abortion of foetus at an early stage, (c) endocrine dysfunction, (d) infection of genital organs.

(a) *Temperamental factors.* Refusal to mate is uncommon in the cow and when it does occur it is worth trying Sepia 200c. This remedy has been used successfully in the mare and bitch in similar circumstances and it will be found to have a beneficial effect on the whole genital tract. Dose: one per week for three weeks.

(b) *Abortion of the foetus at an early stage.* Apart from specific diseases such as Brucellosis and Trichomoniasis, non-specific abortion may also occur. Frequently these abortions take the form of an early discharge and the owner or an attendant may be under the impression that no conception has taken place when the animal comes into season later on. A remedy which has given good results under these circumstances is Viburnum Opulis, which has a good reputation in miscarriage generally. It should be given in 30c potency weekly for three weeks. Other remedies which are also of use are Caulophyllum 30c and Sepia 200c given as for Viburnum.

(c) *Endocrine Dysfunction.* In one or other of its manifestations this is probably the most common breeding irregularity. Examples are:

1. *Sub-oestrus or Silent Heat.* This is frequently encountered in winter and clinical features vary from heifers showing no heat cycles to cows which may go several months without a definite oestrus period showing. Remedies to be considered include:

a) *Sepia 200c.* Should be given as a routine remedy because of its generally tonic effect on ovaries and uterus. Dose: one only.

b) *Pulsatilla 30c.* A very good ovarian remedy sometimes associated with vaginal discharge of a creamy consistency. Dose: one per week for three weeks.

c) *Platina 6c.* Has a beneficial action on ovarian function. There may be uterine discharge of catarrhal material associated with urination, the urine itself having a reddish sediment. Dose: one daily for one week.

d) *Aletris Farinosa 30c.* Appetite is usually in abeyance if this remedy is indicated. There is general uterine atony, and a tendency to prolapse. Occasionally uterine bleeding takes place, the blood being dark and membranous. Dose: one twice weekly for three weeks.

e) *Folliculinum 6c.* The intercurrent use of this nosode may aid the action of other remedies. Dose: one daily for three days.

2. *Anoestrus.* From a study of the five stages of the oestrus cycle, it will be seen that only one – anoestrus – is a departure from the normal state when it persists longer than about eight weeks after parturition. It is of fairly common occurrence. Remedies employed to initiate a new cycle include the following:

a) *Pulsatilla 30c.* Should be given as for Silent Heat. Also after retained placenta.

b) *Calcarea Phosphorica 30c.* When indicated there is usually a profuse leucorrhoea, worse in the morning and sometimes accompanying a vaginitis. Dose: one daily for three days, followed by one every second day for three doses.

c) *Iodum 30c.* This is a good remedy if the ovaries feel small and shrivelled on rectal examination. Suitable for lean animals with good appetite and active temperament. Dose: one daily for ten days.

3. *Cystic ovaries.* Cows as distinct from heifers are principally affected with this abnormality, and the ovaries may contain several cysts. The condition is frequently associated with hyperplasia of the endometrium. Clinical signs are those which appear with irregular heat periods and nymphomania with changes in the shape of the pelvic girdle. Such animals are troublesome to others. The following remedies should be considered:

a) *Apis Mellifica 6c.* This is a useful remedy for dissolving cysts by causing absorption of fluid. Dose: one twice daily for one week.

b) *Murex Purpurea 30c.* A good remedy for nymphomania and for regulating the oestrus cycle. Dose: one dose per week for three weeks.

c) *Natrum Muriaticum 30c.* Indicated when there is an accompanying greenish discharge from the vagina which at the same time feels dry. Dose: one daily for one week.

d) *Colocynthis 6c.* When nymphomania is associated with the presence of multiple small cysts. Signs of abdominal pain are usually present. Dose: one twice daily for one week.

e) *Platina 30c.* Catarrhal vaginitis is often present along with reddish sediment in the urine. A very good ovarian remedy in general. Dose: one three times daily for five days.

f) *Palladium 6c.* If the right ovary alone is affected this remedy could well be indicated. Dose: one twice daily for one week.

g) *Oopherinum 6x.* Ovarian extract frequently brings about resolution of the cyst, if used in low potency. There may be an accompanying skin irritation when this remedy is indicated. Dose: one daily for five days.

h) *Rhododendron 30c.* Also indicated in right ovarian involvement but there are usually accompanying cysts present in the vagina. Dose: one daily for one week.

4. *Persistent Corpus Luteum.* By this we mean the persistence of a functioning corpus luteum in the abscence of pregnancy. It is usually associated with uterine changes, either pyometritis or endometric hyperplasia. Remedies to be considered are:

a) *Folliculinum 6c.* The follicle hormone potentised will be found to be of service in bringing about resolution. Dose: one daily for five days.

b) *Pulsatilla 30c.* Will act on the ovarian tissues generally and will help to restore normal ovary function. Dose: one daily for five days.

c) *Sepia 200c* For regulating the activity of the genital tract and aiding the action of other remedies. Dose: one single dose.

d) *Thuja 6c.* For implication of left ovary particularly. There may be evidence of abdominal pain along left flank. Dose: one twice daily for one week.

5. *Frequent return to service or failure to hold.* When this has its origins in endocrine dysfunction it is usually due to ovulatory failure during an otherwise normal oestrus. It is a frequent cause of infertility. The following remedies will all help in promoting ovulation:

a) *Sepia 200c.* One single dose.

b) *Pulsatilla 30c.* There may be an accompanying vaginal discharge of semi-purulent material. Dose: one weekly for three weeks.

c) *Calcarea Phosphorica 30c.* Useful remedy for younger animals (heifers). Catarrhal vaginal discharge may be present. Dose: as for Pulsatilla.

d) *Iodum 30c.* Indicated when rectal examination reveals a

shrivelled state of ovaries, or if they are small and hard. The animal may be thin with excessive appetite. Dose: as for the previous remedies.

e) *Oopherinum 6x.*   The ovarian extract in potency may be used in conjunction with other remedies. Dose: one daily for five days.

6. *Salpingitis.*   The funnel-shaped arrangement of the junction of the uterine cornua with the oviducts in the bovine favours infection from the uterus. Pyogenic Salpingitis leads to sterility and can be controlled by remedies such as the following:

a) *Hepar Sulphuris 30c.*   Useful in the early stages when inflammation of the oviducts produces symptom of lower abdominal pain. Undue heat and throbbing may be felt on rectal examination. Dose: one every three hours for four doses.

b) *Mercurius Sol 30c.*   A greenish purulent discharge may be present per vaginam, resulting from a pyometritis. The discharge may be blood-stained. Dose: one twice daily for ten days.

c) *Hydrastis 30c.*   This is also a good remedy for pyometritis, the discharge being catarrhal and profuse. Dose: as for Mercurius.

d) *Pulsatilla 30c.*   Bland creamy discharges which may have their origin in retained placenta indicate this remedy. Dose: three time daily for four days.

(d)   *Infection of Genital Organs.*   These include *Puerperal Metritis*, *Vibrio fetus* infection, *Trichomoniasis* and contagious *Vesicular Vaginitis*, to all of which reference has already been made (see pages 71–78).

18. Diseases of Calves

1. Coli-Bacillosis – White Scour. This is an acute infectious disease characterised by prostration accompanying the passage of liquid or semi-liquid faeces with frequent complications of a septicaemic nature, such as pneumonia.

ETIOLOGY. It is generally accepted that one of the many strains of the E. Coli organism is responsible.

As an introduction to the study of Coli-bacillosis, let us examine statements made by the late Dr John Paterson, the eminent homoeopathic physician and microbiologist, whose researches on the Bowel Nosodes opened up new fields in the study of non-lactose fermenting bacteria. In an address to the Rhodanienne Homoeopathic Society, Dr Paterson stated 'It must now be accepted as scientific fact that specific germs in many cases of disease can be isolated and identified, but is it a true conclusion that the specific germ is always the cause of the disease? We must consider the role of the bacterium in nature, because on this we must determine the value one places on bacterial products – oral vaccines and nosodes – in the treatment of disease'.

In the light of the above remarks let us look briefly at the role of the E. Coli organism. Microbiologists are now in general agreement that this bacterium is a harmless saprophyte, and in the normal healthy bowel is considered to be non-pathogenic. The main function of this organism is to break up complex molecules resulting from the digestive process into simpler substances. We see as a result of this observation that E. Coli plays a useful role in the normal, healthy intestinal tract, and where the intestinal mucosa is healthy the organism is non-pathogenic. If, however, the mucosa is affected in any way by changes in the host, the normal balance will be upset and the E. Coli organism may then become pathogenic. This is probably due to a change in its habitat, and possibly also in its biochemic structure. This is an example of a bacterium becoming modified in order to survive. It is important to note that the E. Coli organism is not the primary cause of disease – this originates in the host due to the changes we have noted.

CHIEF CLINICAL SIGNS OF COLI-BACILLOSIS.   Calves may appear normal at birth but quickly show signs of shock, viz. cold muzzle, sub-normal temperature and cold extremities, with rapid weak pulse. This is soon followed by whitish or yellow pasty faeces rapidly becoming liquid, and often preceded by abdominal bloating. The motion has a characteristic sickly odour. Sudden prostration is common and is to be construed as a serious development. An interesting feature is the absence of fever, unusual in a disease associated with bacterial invasion. A frequent sequel is pneumonia due to septicaemic complications.

SUSCEPTIBILITY.   Calves which are deprived of colostrum are particularly at risk, while those bought in from market may show severe symptoms: such animals frequently being susceptible on both counts. Also at risk are calves born in unhygienic surroundings, or being put into infected calving pens. Faulty diet of the dam may contribute, while cold wet weather predisposes calves to illness. All these hazards constitute changes in the host which renders it more susceptible to disease.

TREATMENT.   The following remedies will be found useful according to symptoms and the nature of the diarrhoea.
1. *Aconitum Napellus 6c.*   Should always be given as a preliminary remedy and acts especially well in cases which arise suddenly or as a sequel to exposure to cold wind. Dose: one every one and a half hours for six doses.
2. *Arsenicum Album 30c.*   Frequent watery stools accompanied by straining. The skin around the anus becomes excoriated. The coat is dry and harsh, and has a dehydrated look. Motions tend to have a cadaverous odour, and the patient will drink more than normal if allowed. Restlessness is obvious and the calf shifts position frequently. Dose: one every two hours for four doses.
3. *China Officinalis 30c.*   This remedy is of great value in restoring strength after loss of body fluid. It also has a beneficial effect directly on the gut by helping to alleviate diarrhoea. Dose: one three-hourly for four doses.

4. *Veratrum Album 30c.* With this remedy there is a general appearance of collapse with signs of abdominal pain preceding the onset of diarrhoea. Stools are watery and forcibly evacuated, while body-sweating is present as a rule. The calf is cold and visible mucous membranes may have a bluish tinge. Dose: one every two hours for four doses.

5. *Pulsatilla 30c.* When the remedy is indicated it will be found that the character of the stool changes frequently, e.g. at one stage it may contain a significant amount of mucus while at another time it may be watery. Changeability of symptoms is a keynote of this remedy. Dose: one three times daily for two days.

6. *Carbo Vegetabilis 200c.* Stools are preceded by signs of abdominal colic with flatulence. It is an excellent remedy for helping to revive apparently moribund patients. Such calves should be given generous access to fresh air. Dose: one every hour for four doses.

7. *Pyrogen 1m.* This is one of the most valuable remedies we can employ when septicaemic complications arise, characterised by discrepancies in pulse and temperature, e.g. a sub-normal temperature is usually associated with a rapid pulse. The temperature is usually elevated when Pyrogen is indicated, but this rarely happens in coli-bacillosis unless pneumonia supervenes, when again the remedy may be needed. Calves in need of Pyrogen invariably have a putrid odour. Dose: one every three hours for four doses.

8. *Dulcamara 30c.* A useful remedy if the onset of disease symptoms is associated with exposure to damp. Autumn-born calves are more likely to need this remedy than those born in the spring. Dose: one three times daily for two days.

9. *Camphora 6c.* This is another remedy which is associated with collapsed states. There is extreme coldness of body and mouth while motions may be passed involuntarily. Dose: one every half-hour for six doses.

10. *E. Coli Nosode 30c.* It has been found in practice that the use of this nosode provides rapid relief if not too long delayed. There are various strains of this organism available but the original one, prepared from a human source, has given the most consistent results. Dose: one three times daily for two days.

PREVENTION OF COLI-BACILLOSIS. If the nosode is administered immediately at birth, and again at 24, 48 and 72 hours, it will greatly reduce the chance of infection arising. Calves which do contract scour after being given the nosode prophylactically will be only mildly affected. Where Coli-bacillosis is an established herd problem, this approach should be strengthened by administering the nosode to in-calf cows, giving one dose weekly for the last month of pregnancy.

2. Joint-ill. Omphalophlebitis. Navel ill. This is the name given to the forms of arthritis associated with bacterial invasion of the system attendant on unhygienic surroundings at birth, although it may arise also when proper care is exercised.

ETIOLOGY. Various bacteria are incriminated but the disease is usually associated with strains of E. Coli or Streptococcus species.

SYMPTOMS. There may be a short febrile stage followed by obvious signs of lameness and pain. The joints commonly affected are the hock, stifle and carpus and they become swollen and hot. The animal resents touch. Suppuration of the joint may quickly supervene if the invading bacteria are of the pyogenic type. Swelling and pain of the navel area may also be present but this is not a constant sign.

TREATMENT. The main remedies to be considered are:
1. *Aconitum Napellus 12x.* Will be of useful if the disease is recognised in the early febrile phase. Dose: one every half-hour for four doses.
2. *Bryonia Alba 30c.* Joints are swollen and hot and have a tense stretched feel. Movement aggravates the pain and the animal does not resent pressure on the affected part. Dose: one every two hours for four doses.
3. *Ruta Graveolens 1m.* Will relieve pains associated with inflammation of the surrounding periosteum and tendons, particularly when the carpus is involved. Dose: one every two hours for four doses.
4. *Ledum Palustre 30c.* Joints chiefly affected are shoulder and fetlock. Dose: one three times daily for three days.
5. *Benzoicum Acidum 6c.* Principally for involvement of hock with accompanying swelling and heat in Achilles tendon. Dose: one every three hours for four doses.

6. *Streptococcus 30c.* This Nosode has proved invaluable in practice, its early use obviating the need for subsequent remedies. Dose: one dose three times daily for two days, followed by one dose every second day for three doses.
7. *E. Coli 30c.* If this organism is suspected a course of the Nosode as for streptococcus will probably prove useful.

3. Calf diphtheria. A disease characterised by the presence of necrotic areas in the mouth and throat.

ETIOLOGY. A bacillus named Fusiformis necrophorus is responsible. It is a soil contaminant and is associated with necrosis of various tissues.

SYMPTOMS. There is an initial febrile stage when the organism gains entrance to the system. The first symptom seen is usually salivation accompanying stomatitis. The gums bordering the upper teeth become swollen and a foul smell is noticeable. When the laryngeal area becomes affected there is difficulty in breathing, with coughing and signs of distress. The tip of the tongue may protrude and may be covered by necrotic patches. The infection frequently extends to the lungs precipitating an acute pneumonia.

TREATMENT.
1. *Aconitum Napellus 12x.* Should be given when early feverish signs are present. Dose: one every half-hour for four doses.
2. *Mercurius Solubilis 6c.* For the stage of stomatitis with salivation and swollen throat. Dose: one four times in 24 hours.
3. *Mercurius Corrosivus 200c.* When gums are swollen and purplish in appearance there may be an accompanying looseness of some teeth. Dose: one three times daily for three days.
4. *Mercurius Cyanatus 6c.* The most important remedy when ulceration and necrosis affects the throat, the mucous membrane of which sloughs easily. There may be an associated bleeding from nose. Dose: one three times daily for four days.
5. *Mercurius Iodatus Flavus 6c.* A useful remedy when the right side of the throat and tonsillar area is involved. Necrotic patches are easily detached. Dose: one three times daily for four days.
6. *Mercurius Iodatus Ruber 6c.* For swollen gums and associated throat glands. Salivation is profuse. Inflammatory lesions are worse on the left side. Dose: one three times daily for four days.

7. *Muriaticum Acidum 30c.*   For swollen tongue which protrudes and has deep lesions. Necrotic areas have a brown leathery appearance. Dose: one twice daily for one week.
8. *Tuberculinum Aviare 200c.*   This remedy may prove useful for secondary pneumonia cases. It acts well in the young animal. Dose: one daily for seven days.
9. *Bromium 6c.*   Also useful for the croupous pneumonia which may develop. Spasmodic cough with signs of bronchial congestion and production of mucus. Dose: one three times daily for five days.

4.   Salmonellosis.   This disease may be encountered as an acute septicaemia or as an inflammation of the intestines, sometimes chronic.

ETIOLOGY.   In cattle there are two main species responsible – *S. typhimurium* and *S. dublin.*

SYMPTOMS.   Infection is frequently encountered in calves up to three months. In the septicaemic form calves may show signs of involvement of the central nervous system, such as incoordination and muscular twitching. The most commonly encountered form is the abdominal or enteric which is usually acute. A high temperature – up to 106°F – is followed by excessive watery diarrhoea which may be blood-stained and contain mucus. The smell is foul or putrid and severe straining is occasionally seen. The temperature usually falls once diarrhoea starts. There is lack of appetite but thirst is prominent. Heart rate is increased and accompanied by shallow respirations. Visible mucous membranes are injected or reddened. Occasionally the joints become affected resulting in swelling and arthritis. This usually follows recovery from an acute attack.

TREATMENT.   Septicaemic cases invariably die before treatment can be started but in the other forms the following remedies should be considered:
1. *Aconitum 12x.*   Should if possible be given early in the acute phase. Dose: one every half-hour for four doses.
2. *Arsenicum Album 1m.*   Will help control the watery, foul-smelling diarrhoea. Dose: one every three hours for four doses.

3. *Veratrum Album 30c.* When collapse is threatened and faeces are forcibly evacuated. Dose: one every two hours for six doses.
4. *Pyrogenium 1m.* Indicated in putrid or septic states where there is high temperature alternating with a weak thready pulse. Discharges are extremely offensive. Dose: one every three hours for four doses.
5. *Rhus Toxicodendon 1m.* Where there is pronounced redness of visible mucous membranes. Dose: one twice daily for four days.
6. *Bryonia 30c.* May be useful in arthritis cases where movement aggravates. This remedy should also be useful in controlling respiratory symptoms. Dose: twice daily for three days.
7. *Salmonella Nosode 30c.* This Nosode has been prepared from the two common types associated with calf disease. For treatment one dose should be given three times daily for two days and may profitably be combined with indicated remedies. For prevention, calves should have one dose at birth and repeated at fortnightly intervals for four doses.

5. Coccidiosis. This is a dysenteric disease of calves characterised by the passage of whole blood in the faeces, and affecting calves in any age group. It is most frequently seen in summer and principally associated with insanitary conditions.

ETIOLOGY. A protozoan parasite caused by Eimeria species, the two commonest being E. zurnii and E. bovis. On ingestion the infective stage of the parasite is liberated into the intestine and penetration of the epithelium occurs.

SYMPTOMS. An acute haemorrhagic enteritis is set up confined to the large intestine, after an incubation period of 1–3 weeks. Loss of blood in the early stages is followed by weakness, pallor of visible mucous membranes, anorexia and loss of condition. The dysentery arising is frequently foul-smelling and accompanied by great straining. Pneumonia is a not uncommon complication. Milder outbreaks may contain little or no blood, but persistent diarrhoea is the rule along with a dry coat and unthrifty appearance.

TREATMENT.
1. *Aconitum Napellus 12x.* If seen in the early stages when feverish symptoms are being ushered in. Dose: one every half-hour for four doses.

2. *Arsenicum Album 1m.* This remedy should prove valuable both in the acute dysenteric stage and also for milder cases showing loss of condition with dry coat and unthrifty appearance. Dose: in acute cases one dose every two hours for five doses. In milder cases one dose per day for one week.

3. *Ipecacuanha 30c.* This is an important remedy for this particular condition. Not only is it a good anti-haemorrhagic remedy in its own right but it appears to have a specific action on the intestines in the presence of protozoa. Dose: one dose three times daily for four days.

4. *Mercurius Corrosivus 200c.* A very useful remedy to control dysentery accompanied by the presence of mucus and much straining. Dose: one four times daily for two days.

5. *Cinchona 6c.* This remedy will help restore strength after loss of blood. Dose: one three times daily for three days.

6. *Veratrum Album 30c.* For milder cases showing persistent diarrhoea of an explosive type with threatened weakness and collapse. Dose: one three times daily for two days.

7. *Sycotic Co. 6c.* This Bowel Nosode may be given once daily for three days as an aid to above remedies. It acts selectively on the mucous membrane of the intestines.

6. Disorders of Calcium Metabolism. Such disorders usually take the form of a combined calcium and phosphorus deficiency. This is more common than shortage of vitamin D and may be seen in calves which have received an inadequate intake of milk, together with an excess of cereal grains.

SYMPTOMS. These are most commonly seen in calves which put on weight quickly and take the form of deformities in the joints, especially the knees, which become stiff and swollen, and the junctions of the ribs at the sternal cage. The gait becomes stiff and the limbs may show weakness such as bending. Appetite may be indifferent in advanced cases and there is also a tendency to fracture of various bones, especially the long bones, which remain thin, and the ribs.

TREATMENT. The carbonate and phosphate of calcium are the remedies of choice according to type.

1. *Calcarea Carbonica 30c.* This is more suitable for the heavy fleshy calf which has fed well on inadequate food. The animal may sweat easily and be lethargic. Dose: one twice daily for two weeks.

2. *Calcarea Phosphorica 30c.* This is the more commonly employed remedy combining as it does the Ca. and P. factors. Dose: as above.

3. *Symphytum 6x.* If fractures are threatened or have actually taken place on advanced cases. Dose: one three times daily for one week.

PREVENTION.   As well as adequate and proper food, calves may be given Calcarea Phosph. 30c as a mineral additive. This will ensure proper calcium and phosphorus metabolism. One dose twice weekly should be sufficient.

7. Copper Deficiency.   This particular mineral deficiency may take the form of a scour in calves over two months of age, or it may be seen as a pining condition unassociated with scouring.

SYMPTOMS.   Calves which show scouring associated with copper deficiency are invariably stunted and frequently develop intercurrent infections. The more frequently encountered deficiency takes the form of a pining condition and is seen most often in beef rearing herds in early summer when calves and their dams have been turned out to grass. Unthriftiness is followed by weak movements and the coat becomes harsh and dry. Black cattle show loss or discolouration of hair around the eyes giving a 'spectacled' appearance which is almost pathognomonic of the condition. Red-coated calves become yellowish or rust-coloured. Copper deficiency is commonly seen in lime-free and marginal ground.

TREATMENT.   Different preparations of copper are employed according to symptoms displayed.

1. *Cuprum Aceticum 6c.*   A useful remedy for scouring calves. The abdomen is usually tympanitic prior to evacuation. Stools may be dark with blood-stained mucus. Animal is generally weak and trembling. Dose: one every two hours for four doses, followed by one twice daily for three days.

2. *Cuprum Arsenicosum 30c.*   A useful remedy for the less acute scouring calf showing slimy diarrhoea on first going out to grass. There may be increased thirst. Walking produces tremulous movements. Dose: one three times daily for three days.
3. *Cuprum Metallicum 1m.*   This is the form generally employed in pining outbreaks unassociated with scouring. It will greatly alleviate the cramping gait and restore normal colouration to the coat. Dose: one daily for fourteen days.

8.   Bloat Tympany.   Rumenal bloat is occasionally seen in young calves which are fed whole milk or milk substitutes for long periods.

SYMPTOMS.   The left side of the calf becomes distended due to the accumulation of gas in the rumen. This can arise very quickly. Slower cases develop over a longer period and symptoms of tympany may be intermittent, gas accumulating over a period of days. The calf quickly becomes distressed and appetite is in abeyance.

TREATMENT.   The main remedies are as follows and should be given promptly.
1. *Colchinum 200c.*   Probably the most effective remedy in acute cases. Dose: one every fifteen minutes for four or five doses.
2. *Nux Vomica 1m.*   For less acute cases which may arise from the administration of too much food rather than the wrong sort. Dose: one every half-hour for four doses.
3. *Lycopodium 1m.*   A useful remedy for the more chronic case in the poorly fed calf. Dose: one twice daily for one week.
4. *Baryta Carbonica 6c.*   Also useful for the less acute case in the younger calf. The abdomen will feel tense and full. Dose: one three times daily for four days.
5. *Carbo Vegetabilis 200c.*   For use in those cases accompanied by bowel rumblings and arising immediately after a meal. Dose: one every half-hour for five doses.

9.   Infectious Keratitis – New Forest Disease.   This commonly occuring condition in young animals is seen principally in the summer months, although winter outbreaks do occur among calves housed in overcrowded insanitary conditions. In summer spread is hastened by flies.

ETIOLOGY. Bacteria of the Moraxella group are thought to be implicated but viruses may also play a part.

SYMPTOMS. The condition may attack one or both eyes. After an incubation period of about one week, lachrymation arises. The conjunctivae become reddened and inflamed. A white opaque spot develops on the cornea and rapidly increases in size until it covers the entire cornea, leading eventually to ulceration. Secondary infection by pyogenic bacteria is common in neglected cases and leads to the development of ophthalmia with resulting purulent discharges.

TREATMENT. It is essential that treatment be instituted as rapidly as possible owing to the virulence of the infection.
1. *Aconitum 12x.* Should be given immediately any trouble is suspected. The animal at this stage may be listless with slightly inflamed eye. Dose: one every half-hour for five doses.
2. *Kali Hydriodicum 200c.* A useful remedy for the early stages when the eye shows lachrymation and reddened lids. Dose: one three times daily for four days.
3. *Silicea 200c.* This is the remedy of choice when corneal opacity has set in. It will aid resorption of scar tissue. Dose: one daily for seven days.
4. *Acidum Nitricum 200c.* If corneal ulceration has started this remedy may bring about speedy resolution. Dose: one twice daily for five days.
5. *Argentum Nitricum 30c.* If ophthalmia is threatening with purulent discharge beginning. Dose: one three times daily for one week.
6. *Cineraria 3x.* Also a useful remedy for corneal opacity. It could be combined with silicea for this purpose. Dose: one three times daily for one week.
7. *Calendula, Hypericum and Cineraria Lotions.* May be used externally in a dilution of 1/10 and the eye bathed frequently.

PREVENTION. A nosode exists and should be given to all calves at risk. One dose for three consecutive days should be followed by a monthly dose for three months.

10. Leptospirosis. This disease of calves is usually seen in winter, the source of infection being food contaminated by rat urine.

Once an animal is infected, the disease can spread directly from calf to calf.

ETIOLOGY.   A bacterium named *Leptospira icterohaemorrhagica*. This parasite is harboured by rats and spread through the urine.

SYMPTOMS.   The younger age group are more prone to infection. There is an incubation period of up to one week, followed by a rise in temperature up to 107°F. Dullness and inappetance occur along with rapid loss of condition which may progress to emaciation. Jaundice in varying degrees is usually present, being most prominent in the eyes and gums. Severe cases may end fatally but normally the course is sub-acute.

TREATMENT.   At the first sign of jaundice the following remedies should be considered:
1. *Aconitum 12x.*   For the early invasive stage when temperature is starting to rise, if noticed in time. Dose: one every half-hour for five doses.
2. *Crotalus Horridus 1m.*   Probably the most important remedy to be considered. Has a direct effect on the haemolytic jaundice syndrome. Dose: one every two hours for five doses as early as possible.
3. *Berberis Vulgaris 30c.*   A useful remedy for the less acute case. It has a specific action on the liver and will aid the function of that gland. Dose: one three times daily for five days.
4. *Phosphorus 1m.*   Useful also in the more acute case. Will help prevent damage to liver cells. Dose: one twice daily for one week.
5. *Lycopodium 1m.*   Useful remedy for the convalescent stage when emaciation or loss of condition is apparent. Will restore liver function and aid digestion. Dose: one per day for one week.

11.   Hyperkeratosis.   This skin condition is associated with an interference with the conversion of the pigment carotene into Vitamin A. External mechanical influences play a part.

SYMPTOMS.   Early signs include lachrymation, salivation and disinclination to feed. Loss of condition follows, while the mucous membranes of the mouth and tongue become eroded into large patches. This represents the acute phase of the condition. Chronic cases show skin changes chiefly confined to the neck where the hair is lost and the skin becomes dry, thickened and wrinkled. These skin changes may extend down between the fore-legs.

TREATMENT. Different remedies may be needed according to the phase of the condition.

1. *Kali Hydriodicum 200c.* Valuable in the early stages showing lachrymation and inappetance. Dose: one twice daily for four days.
2. *Acidum Nitricum 200c.* Will be of service in treating the mouth and tongue lesions. Dose: one three times daily for four days.
3. *Kali Arsenicum 30c.* This remedy is useful in the more chronic stage where skin lesions have taken place. It has a most beneficial effect on the skin. Dose: one daily for two weeks.
4. *Graphites 6c.* Also useful for the chronic stage. Will control skin inflammation and oozings which tend to occur in the folds of thickened skin. Dose: one three times daily for five days.
5. *Hydrocotyle 6c.* A very useful remedy for skin proliferation with thickening of epidermis. Dose: one three times daily for four days, followed by a daily dose of 200c.
6. *Lycopodium 1m.* This remedy will help constitutionally. It has a beneficial action on the liver which is frequently affected. Dose: one daily for ten days.
7. *Bacillinum 200c.* The intercurrent use of this nosode may help in treatment. A single dose should suffice.

12. Enzootic Pneumonia. Virus Pneumonia. This is a highly infectious respiratory disease, affecting chiefly the two- to eight-month age group.

ETIOLOGY. Various viruses are implicated; bacterial involvement is considered to be secondary.

SYMPTOMS. There is an initial temperature rise up to 107°F, or occasionally a sub-normal temperature may occur. Difficult breathing is soon evident accompanied by a short, dry, hacking cough. The laboured breathing may compel the calf to open its mouth in an attempt to increase inhalation. Exertion or handling causes distress. Rasping sounds are heard on auscultation. Nasal and oral discharge may be present, the former at first watery, but later becoming purulent or blood-stained. Frequently it is rust-coloured. Very acute cases may show no discharge. In chronic cases emphysema and lung abscesses develop and the calf remains unthrifty with stunted growth.

TREATMENT. The animal should be confined to a cool, well-ventilated box. The following remedies should be considered.

1. *Aconitum 12x.* For the early febrile stage. Dose: one every half-hour for four doses.
2. *Antimonium Tartaricum 1m.* Moist cough indicates this remedy. Frothy mucus may be seen. Dose: one every two hours for four doses.
3. *Bryonia 30c.* When pleurisy is suspected. Cough is dry and hard. The animal prefers rest and is worse on motion. Dose: one three times daily for one week.
4. *Arsenicum Album 1m.* The calf is restless and symptoms are aggravated toward midnight. Drinking is frequent and the patient seeks cool places. Dose: one every two hours for four doses.
5. *Drosera 9c.* Spasmodic cough with quick breathing. Cough appears to come from the throat or upper trachea. Dose: one three times daily for five days.
6. *Phosphorus 1m.* Indicated when solidification of lung tissue has set in. Very acute cases may need this remedy. Dose: one every half-for five doses.
7. *Rhus Toxicodendron 1m* For cases showing heat and redness of buccal mucosa and hairless parts of the skin. Animal may prefer to move about. Dose: one three times daily for three days.
8. *Lobelia Inflata 200c.* A useful remedy in chronic cases showing emphysema. Dose: one twice daily for two weeks.
9. *Ammonium Causticum 200c.* Also useful in emphysema. Digestive upsets are usually present. Dose: one twice daily for one week.

PREVENTION. A Nosode has been prepared from the commoner viruses implicated. Calves should be given one dose at birth and repeated weekly for four weeks.

13. Mucosal Disease. This disease, also called Bovine Virus Diarrhoea, is characterised by ulceration of the mucous membranes of the alimentary and respiratory tracts.

ETIOLOGY. A specific virus is responsible.

SYMPTOMS. An initial febrile phase produces a temperature rise which may be as much as 108°F. Pulse rate is increased and accompanies a discharge of clear mucus which soon becomes mucopurulent. Within 48 hours the mucous membranes of the nasal passages become bright pink and small shallow ulcers develop on the muzzle which assumes a bronze-red appearance. These ulcers also appear inside the lips and on the hard palate. Salivation accompanies these developments. Diarrhoea soon sets in which becomes profuse leading to dehydration. Respiratory involvement is evidenced by rapid breathing and coughing. In young calves there may be no signs except the appearance of the shallow ulcers on the gums and muzzle and the bronzed appearance of the latter. The buccal mucosa in these cases is bright red.

TREATMENT.
1. *Aconitum 30c.* Four doses at half-hourly intervals should be given at the initial febrile stage if this can be noticed.
2. *Acidum Nitricum 200c.* This remedy has given good results in cases where ulceration develops around the mouth and nose and also on the lower rectum. Give one dose night and morning for one week.
3. *Rhus Toxicodendron 6c.* When the appearance of the buccal mucosa is fiery red this remedy may produce good results. It will also limit the extension of mouth lesions. Dose: one thrice daily for five days.
4. *Natrum Muriaticum 6c.* When the main signs are the appearance of the small shallow ulcers on the gums and papillae this remedy may be of value. It is more suitable for the milder case. Dose: one thrice daily for one week.
5. *Arsenicum Album 1m.* Should help control diarrhoea which will be watery and blood-stained when this remedy is indicated. Dose: one twice daily for four days.
6. *Cuprum Arsenicum 6c.* Slimy diarrhoea with respiratory involvement indicates this remedy. Dose: one twice daily for four days.
7. *Kali Bichromicum 200c.* Ulcers develop a punched-out look and have a yellow base. Nasal discharge of yellow mucus is present. Dose: one daily for seven days.
8. *Mercurius Corrosivus 200c.* Salivation accompanies a slimy blood-stained diarrhoea with great tenesmus. The ulcers develop

a septic look with dirty gums. Secondary infection may lead to this state. Dose: one thrice daily for two days followed by one daily for three days.

9. *Cinchona 6c.* This remedy will help control the weakness accompanying dehydration and may be given concurrently with other remedies. Dose: one thrice daily for two days.

10. *Drosera 9c.* A useful remedy for controlling coughing and respiratory involvement generally. Dose: one thrice daily for five days.

14. Calf Hypomagnesaemia. This may be seen under varying systems of management and is common to both beef and dairy animals. It may be associated with a very high milk intake, and as the amounts of magnesium excreted in the milk may vary from cow to cow, the incidence in any one herd may vary accordingly. It is unusual to encounter this trouble in calves under two months of age.

CLINICAL SIGNS. The calf is unduly excitable and this very often accompanies changes in the manner in which the head is carried; e.g. there may be retraction of the head together with restless movements. The feet are lifted high with an exaggerated motion producing a spastic form of movement. All reflexes are pronounced, particularly tendon reflexes. Convulsions may follow a latent state of muscle tetany along with a quickening of the heart's action and laboured respiration.

TREATMENT. Injections of magnesium sulphate are normally effective, but to supplement these, the following remedies will be found useful in preventing relapse and minimising damage to the central nervous system.

1. *Belladonna 1m.* A valuable remedy for controlling convulsions and preventing brain damage. Pupils are usually dilated and pulse is full and bounding. Dose: one every half-hour for four doses.

2. *Stramonium 200c.* With this remedy there is a tendency to fall forwards. Tetany of isolated groups of muscles occurs with twitching of tendons. Dose: one every hour for four doses.

3. *Cicuta Virosa 30c.* For those cases where retraction of the head is the principle symptom; there is also a spasmodic condition of the neck muscles. Dose: one three times daily for three days.

4. *Magnesium Phosphoricum 30c.* The administration of magnesium in potency helps stabilise the element in the system. This is a valuable attribute of the potentised remedy, when we remember that in allopathic injectable form it can quickly be excreted. It can profitably be combined with calcarea phosphorica in the same potency as frequently there is disturbance to the calcium metabolism at the same time. Dose: one dose of each twice daily for three days given in alternation.

15. Muscular Dystrophy. Vitamin E Deficiency. This condition may be encountered in suckling herds when the cows have been wintered on an inadequate diet being deprived of a proper intake of minerals and vitamins. It can occur indoors but is more usually seen when calves are turned out for the first time in late spring. It normally attacks calves up to three months of age but may be met with less often in the older calf.

CLINICAL SIGNS. The musculo-skeletal system is involved resulting in a picture of stiffness and/or paralysis if the limbs are affected and rapid breathing suggestive of pneumonia if the disease attacks the inter-costal muscles. Any muscle or group of muscles may be attacked including the heart muscle when sudden deaths may take place. Affected limbs look swollen and feel spongy.

TREATMENT. The administration of Vitamin E is normally effective but this should be supplemented by the following remedies according to symptoms.
1. *Curare 6c.* For general muscular weakness and also for those cases showing respiratory distress such as rapid breathing. The animal resents pressure on the chest wall. Dose: one thrice daily for one week.
2. *Cuprum Metallicum 1m.* For stiffness and spasm of groups of muscles which may feel rubbery or hard. Dose: one daily for one week.
3. *Conium 30c.* When the condition affects the hind-limbs mainly. The animal may make attempts to rise and appear sound in the fore-limbs. Dose: one three times daily for three days. It may be necessary to follow on with higher potencies.

16. Parasitic Bronchitis – Husk or Hoose. Although this condition can also affect adult animals it is included in the calf section as being mainly associated with young stock. Acute and chronic forms are recognised and the disease is encountered most frequently in summer and early autumn.

ETIOLOGY. *Dictyocaulus viviparus*, a nematode worm is the causal agent, infective larvae being swallowed while the animal is at pasture.

SYMPTOMS. In the acute form coughing is the first noticeable sign and is usually present in a group of animals. The cough is generally husky and the patient extends the neck in a characteristic manner with a protrusion of the tongue. There is nearly always an abundance of froth around the mouth. Signs of respiratory distress are soon evident such as laboured breathing especially on exertion and in severe cases this may be the most prominent symptom, coughing frequently being absent. On auscultation crepitant sounds are heard.

Pulmonary emphysema is the chief accompaniment of the chronic form together with loss of condition, dry staring coat and pallor of visible mucous membranes. The emphysema is a sequel to pneumonia which is always associated with husk.

TREATMENT. Modern anthelmintics are profitably employed in treatment, but the following homoeopathic remedies will be found useful as supplementary agents and will hasten resolution of damaged lung tissue.

1. *Antimonium Tartaricum 30c.* Where there is an abundance of froth together with an excess of mucus producing a frequent moist cough. Mucus may be heard rattling in the chest. Coughing spasm may be worse at night. Dose: one three times daily for five days.

2. *Apis Mellifica 30c.* This is a useful remedy to control the oedema which affects the lung tissue. It can profitably be combined with other remedies. Dose: one every three hours for four doses.

3. *Ammonium Carbonicum 30c.* A useful remedy when pneumonic symptoms are worse in the right lung and the disease accompanies wet chilly weather. The cough is less wet than with *Antimonium Tartaricum.* Dose: one three times daily for four days.

4. *Antimonium Arsenicum 30c.* This remedy is more useful when the left lung is mainly involved and when there is evidence of emphysema. Coughing is worse when the animal is lying down. A valuable remedy in chronic states. Dose: one thrice daily for five days followed by reduced dosage of a higher potency.
5. *Bryonia Alba 6c.* When this remedy is indicated the animal is better at rest and pressure over the chest area relieves the symptoms. The cough is usually dry. Dose: one three times daily for four days.
6. *Arsenicum Album 1m.* For animals with dry staring coats and extreme restlessness. Coughing produces a thick tenacious mucus. There is frequent drinking of small quantities of water. Exposure to draughts or cold air excites the cough and symptoms generally are worse after midnight. Dose: one twice daily for five days.
7. *Arsenicum Iodatum 6c.* A valuable remedy for chronic states with symptoms aggravated by cold and relieved by warmth. The animal is usually worse lying down and finds breathing easier in the standing position. Dose: one three times daily for five days.

PREVENTION OF HUSK. A reliable Nosode exists which has been well proved in practice. Susceptible animals should be given one dose at two months of age, followed by another one month later. This Nosode has been developed from suspensions of contaminated material containing Dictyocaulus viviparus.

Materia Medica

Abies Canadensis. Hemlock Spruce. N.O. Coniferae
The ∅ is made from the fresh bark and young buds.

This plant has an affinity for mucous membranes generally and that of the stomach in particular, producing a catarrhal gastritis. Impairment of liver function occurs leading to flatulence and deficient bile-flow. Appetite is increased and hunger may be ravenous. It is chiefly used as a digestive remedy.

Aconitum Napellus. Monkshood. N.O. Ranunculaceae.
In the preparation of the ∅ the entire plant is used as all parts contain aconitine the active principle.

This plant has an affinity for serous membranes and muscular tissues leading to functional disturbances. There is sudden involvement and tension in all parts. This remedy should be used in the early stages of all feverish conditions where there is sudden appearance of symptoms which may also show an aggravation when any extreme of temperature takes place. Predisposing factors which may produce a drug picture calling for aconitum include shock, operation and exposure to cold dry winds, or dry heat. It could be of use in puerperal conditions showing sudden involvement with peritoneal complications.

Aesculus Hippocastanum. Horse Chestnut. N.O. Sapindaceae.
The ∅ is prepared from the fruit with capsule.

The main affinity of this plant is with the lower bowel producing a state of venous congestion. There is a general slowing down of the digestive and circulatory systems, the liver and portal action becoming sluggish. This is associated with a tendency to dry stools. It is a useful remedy in hepatic conditions with venous congestion affecting the general circulation and it also has a place in the treatment of congestive chest conditions.

Agaricus Muscarius. Fly Agaric. N.O. Fungi.
The ⌀ is prepared from the fresh fungus.

Muscarin is the best known toxic compound of several which are found in this fungus. Symptoms of poisoning are generally delayed from anything up to twelve hours after ingestion. The main sphere of action is on the central nervous system producing a state of vertigo and delirium followed by sleepiness. There are four recognised stages of cerebral excitement. Viz: 1. Slight stimulation. 2. Intoxication with mental excitement accompanied by twitching. 3. Delirium. 4. Depression with soporific tendency. These actions determine its use in certain conditions affecting the central nervous system, e.g. cerebro-cortical necrosis and meningitis, which may accompany severe attacks of hypomagnesaemia. Tympanitic conditions with flatus may respond favourably while it also has a place as a rheumatic remedy and in the treatment of some forms of muscular cramp.

Aletris Farinosa. Star Grass. N.O. Haemodoraceae.
The ⌀ is prepared from the root.

This plant has an affinity with the female genital tract, especially the uterus and is used mainly as an anti-abortion remedy and in the treatment of uterine discharges and also in silent heat in animals which may show an accompanying loss of appetite.

Allium Cepa. Onion. N.O. Liliaceae.
The ⌀ is prepared from the whole plant.

A picture of coryza with acrid nasal discharge and symptoms of laryngeal discomfort is associated with this plant. It could be indicated in the early stages of most catarrhal conditions producing the typical coryza.

Ammonium Carbonicum. Ammonium Carbonate.
This salt is used as a solution in distilled water from which the potencies are prepared.

It is primarily used in respiratory affections especially when there is an accompanying swelling of associated lymph glands. Emphysema, pulmonary oedema and fog fever are thoracic conditions which may be helped by this remedy. It is also useful in digestive upsets and may promote rumenal activity in sluggish states.

Ammonium Causticum. Hydrate of Ammonia.
Potencies are again prepared from a solution in distilled water.

This salt has a similar but more pronounced action on mucous membranes to that of the carbonate producing ulcerations on these surfaces. It is also a powerful cardiac stimulant. Mucosal disease in calves may call for its use; also respiratory conditions showing severe involvement of the lungs such as fog fever. There is usually an excess of mucus with moist cough when this remedy is indicated.

Antimonium Arsenicosum. Arsenate of Antimony.
Potencies are prepared from trituration of the dried salt dissolved in distilled water or alcohol.

This salt possesses a selective action on the lungs especially the upper left area and is used mainly in the treatment of emphysema and long-standing pneumonias. Coughing, if present, is worse on eating and the animal prefers to stand rather than lie down.

Antimonium Crudum. Sulphide of Antimony.
Potencies prepared from trituration of the dried salt.

This substance exerts a strong influence on the stomach and skin producing conditions which are aggravated by heat. This remedy in cattle practice is used mainly in pustular or eczematous conditions, e.g. cow pox and if given early will prevent complications. Any vesicular skin condition should be influenced favourably.

Antimonium Tartaricum. Tartar Emetic.
Trituration of the dried salt is the source of potencies.

Respiratory symptoms predominate with this drug, affections being accompanied by the production of excess mucus, although expectoration is difficult. The main action being on the respiratory system, we should expect this remedy to be beneficial in conditions such as broncho-pneumonia and pulmonary oedema, e.g. in fog fever. Ailments requiring this remedy frequently show an accompanying drowsiness and lack of thirst. In pneumonic states the edges of the eyes may be covered with mucus.

Apis Mellifica. Bee Venom.
The ⌀ is prepared from the entire insect and also from the venom diluted with alcohol.

The poison of the bee acts on cellular tissue causing oedema and swelling. The production of oedema anywhere in the system may lead to a variety of acute and chronic conditions. Considering the well documented evidence of its sphere of action affecting all tissues and mucous membranes, we should consider this remedy in conditions showing oedematous swellings. Synovial swellings of joints may respond to its use and it has proved of value as an accessory remedy in the treatment of joint-ill in calves if given early. Respiratory conditions showing an excess of pulmonary fluid or oedema, e.g. fog fever, have been treated successfully with this remedy, while it has also been used to good effect in the treatment of cystic ovaries. All ailments are aggravated by heat and are thirstless.

Argentum Nitricum. Silver Nitrate.
This remedy is prepared by trituration of the salt and subsequent dissolving in alcohol or distilled water.

It produces incoordination of movement causing trembling in various parts. It has an irritant effect on mucous membranes producing a free-flowing muco-purulent discharge. Red blood cells are affected, anaemia being caused by their destruction. Its sphere of action makes it a useful remedy in eye conditions, e.g. in New Forest disease.

Arnica Montana. Leopard's Bane. N.O. Compositae.
The ∅ is prepared from the whole fresh plant.

The action of this plant upon the system is practically synonymous with a state resulting from injuries or blows. It is known as the 'Fall Herb' and is used mainly for wounds and injuries where the skin remains unbroken. It has a marked affinity with blood-vessels leading to dilation, stasis and increased permeability. Thus various types of haemorrhage can occur. It reduces shock when given in potency and should be given routinely before and after surgical interference when it will also help control bleeding. Given after parturition it will hasten recovery of bruised tissue, while given during pregnancy at regular intervals, it will help promote normal easy parturition.

Arsenicum Album. Arsenic Trioxide.
This remedy is prepared by trituration and subsequent dilution.

It is a deep acting remedy and acts on every tissue of the body and its characteristic and definite symptoms make its use certain in many ailments. Discharges are acrid and burning and symptoms are relieved by heat. It is of use in many skin conditions associated with dryness, scaliness and itching. Coli-bacillosis and coccidiosis are conditions which may call for its use. It could also have a role to play in some forms of pneumonia when the patient may show a desire for small quantities of water and symptoms becoming worse towards midnight.

Arsenicum Iodatum. Iodide of Arsenic.

Potencies are prepared from the triturated salt dissolved in distilled water.

When discharges are persistently irritating and corrosive, this remedy may prove more beneficial than arsen. alb. The mucous membranes become red, swollen and oedematous, especially in the respiratory sphere. This remedy is frequently called for in bronchial and pneumonic conditions which are at the convalescent stage or in those ailments which have not responded satisfactorily to seemingly indicated remedies.

Baryta Carbonica. Barium Carbonate.

Potencies are prepared from trituration of the salt dissoved in distilled water.

The action of this salt produces symptoms and conditions more usually seen in old and very young subjects and should be remembered as a useful remedy for certain conditions of calves affecting the respiratory system especially.

Belladonna. Deadly Nightshade. N.O. Solanaceae.

The ∅ is prepared from the whole plant at flowering.

This plant produces a profound action on every part of the central nervous system causing a state of excitement and active congestion. The effect also on the skin, glands and vascular system is constant and specific. One of the main guiding symptoms in prescribing is the presence of a full bounding pulse in any feverish condition which may or may not accompany excitable states. The acute form of mastitis seen shortly after parturition may respond well to its use when the udder is hot and tense and swollen. Another guiding symptom is dilation of pupils. In conditions such as hypomagnesaemia and violent forms of milk fever it is useful in preventing damage to the central nervous system.

Bellis Perennis. Daisy. N.O. Compositae.
The ∅ is prepared from the whole fresh plant.

The main action of this little flower is on the muscular tissues of blood vessels producing a state of venous congestion. Systemic muscles become heavy leading to a halting type of gait suggestive of pain. This is a useful remedy to aid recovery of tissues injured during cutting or after operation. Sprains and bruises in general come within its sphere of action and it should be kept in mind as an adjunct remedy along with arnica. Given post-partum it will hasten resolution of bruised tissue and enable the pelvic area to recover tone in a very short time.

Benzoicum Acidum. Benzoic Acid.
Potencies are prepared from gum benzoin which is triturated and dissolved in alcohol.

The most outstanding feature of this remedy relates to the urinary system producing changes in the colour and odour of the urine, which becomes dark red and aromatic with uric acid deposits. It is infrequently used in cattle practice, but may have a place in the treatment of some kidney and bladder conditions.

Berberis Vulgaris. Barberry. N.O. Berberidaceae.
The ∅ is prepared from the bark of the root.

This shrub of wide distribution has an affinity with most tissues. Symptoms which it produces are liable to alternate violently, e.g. feverish conditions with thirst can quickly give way to prostration without any desire for water. It acts forcibly on the venous system producing especially pelvic engorgements. The chief ailments which come within its sphere of action are those connected with liver and kidney leading to catarrhal inflammation of bile ducts and kidney pelvis. Jaundice frequently attends such conditions. Haematuria and cystitis may occur. In all these conditions there is an accompanying sacral weakness and tenderness over the loins.

Beryllium. The Metal.
Trituration and subsequent dissolving in alcohol produces the tincture from which the potencies are prepared.

This remedy is used mainly in respiratory conditions where the leading symptom is difficult breathing on slight exertion and which is out of proportion to clinical findings. Coughing and emphysema are usually present. This is a useful remedy in virus pneumonia, both acute and chronic forms, where symptoms are few while the animal is resting, but become pronounced on movement. It is a deep acting remedy and should not be used below 30c potency.

Borax. Sodium Biborate.
Potencies are prepared from trituration of the salt dissolved in distilled water.

This salt produces gastro-intestinal irritation with mouth symptoms of salivation and ulceration. With most complaints there is fear of downward motion. The specific action of this substance on the epithelium of the mouth, tongue and buccal mucosa determines its use as a remedy which will control such conditions as vesicular stomatitis and allied diseases, e.g. mucosal disease.

Bothrops Lanceolatus. Yellow Viper.
Potencies are prepared from solution of the venom in glycerine.

This poison is associated with haemorrhages and subsequent rapid coagulation of blood. Septic involvement takes place as a rule and this is, therefore, a useful remedy in septic states showing haemorrhagic tendencies. Gangrenous conditions of the skin may respond to it.

Bromium. Bromine. The Element.
Potencies are prepared from solutions in distilled water.

Bromine is found in combination with iodine in the ash when seaweed is burned, and also in sea water. It acts chiefly on the mucous membrane of the respiratory tract, especially the upper trachea causing laryngeal spasm. This is a useful remedy for croup-like cough accompanied by rattling of mucus. Its indication in respiratory ailments is related to symptoms being aggravated on inspiration. It may be of use also in those conditions which arise from overexposure to heat.

Bryonia Alba. White Bryony. Wild Hop. N.O. Cucurbitaceae.
The ⊘ is prepared from the root before flowering takes place.

This important plant produces a glucoside which is capable of bringing on severe purgation. The plant itself exerts its main action on epithelial tissues and serous and synovial membranes. Some mucous surfaces are also affected producing an inflammatory response resulting in a fibrinous or serous exudate. This in turn leads to dryness of the affected tissue with later effusions into synovial cavities. Movement of the parts is interfered with and this leads to one of the main indications for its use, viz. all symptoms are worse from movement, the animal preferring to lie still. Pressure over affected areas relieves symptoms. This remedy may be extremely useful in treating the many respiratory conditions met with, especially pleurisy where the above symptom picture is seen. It is of use in some forms of mastitis where the udder remains hard after initial inflammation has died down.

Cactus Grandiflorus. Night-Blooming Cereus. N.O. Cactaceae.
The ⌀ is prepared from young stems and flowers.

The active principle of this plant acts on circular muscle fibres and has a marked affinity for the cardio-vascular system. It is mainly confined to the treatment of valvular disease, but it may also be of service in some conditions showing a haemorrhagic tendency. It has a limited use in cattle practice.

Calcarea Carbonica. Carbonate of Lime.
Trituration of the salt in alcohol or weak acid produces the solution from which potencies are prepared. The crude substance is found in the middle layer of the Oyster shell.

This calcareous substance produces a lack of tone and muscular weakness with muscle spasm affecting both voluntary and involuntary muscles. Calcium is excreted quickly from the system and the intake of calcium salts does not ensure against conditions which may need the element prepared in the homoeopathic manner. Calc. carb. is a strong costitutional remedy causing impaired nutrition, and animals which need potentised calcium show a tendency to eat strange objects. It is of value in the treatment of skeletal disorders of young animals and in the older animal suffering form osteomalacia. Sessile warts on the teats of heifers come within this sphere of action. As a prophylactic remedy it is used in combination with magnesium and phosphorus to prevent metabolic conditions, such as Milk Fever and hypomagnesaemia.

Calcarea Fluorica. Fluorspar. Fluoride of Lime.
Potencies are prepared from trituration of the salt with subsequent dilution in distilled water.

Crystals of this substance are found in the Haversian canals of bone. This increases the hardness, but in excess produces brittleness. It also occurs in tooth enamel and in the epidermis of the skin. Affinity with all these tissues may lead to the establishment of exostoses and glandular enlargements. It is in addition a powerful vascular remedy. The special sphere of action of this remedy lies in its relation to bone lesions especially exostoses. Both actinomycosis and actinobacillosis may benefit from its use.

Calcarea Phosphorica. Phosphate of Lime.
Potencies are prepared from trituration and subsequent dilution, from adding dilute phosphoric acid to lime water.

This salt has an affinity with tissues which are concerned with growth and the repair of cells. Assimilation may be difficult because of impaired nutrition and delayed development. Brittleness of bone is a common feature. This is a remedy of special value in the treatment of musculo-skeletal disorders of young stock. It may be indicated in some forms of infertility and also as a constitutional remedy for calves suffering from scour.

Calendula Officinalis. Marigold. N.O. Compositae.
The ⌀ is prepared from leaves and flowers.

Applied locally to open wounds and indolent ulcers this remedy will be found to be one of the most reliable healing agents we have. It will rapidly bring about resolution of tissue promoting healthy granulation. It should be used as a 1/10 dilution in warm water. It is helpful in treating contused wounds of the eyes and it can be combined with hypericum when treating open wounds involving damage to nerves.

Camphora. Camphor. N.O. Lauraceae.
Potencies are prepared from a solution of the gum in rectified spirit.

This substance produces a state of collapse with weakness and failing pulse. There is icy coldness of the entire body. It has a marked relationship to muscles and fasciae. Certain forms of scour will benefit from this remedy, viz. those forms accompanied by collapse and extreme coldness of body surfaces. Any form of enteritis showing exhaustion and collapse may require this remedy. It may be needed in disease caused by salmonella species.

Cantharis. Spanish Fly.
The ⌀ is prepared by trituration of the insect with subsequent dilution in alcohol.

The poisonous substances contained in this insect attack, particularly, the urinary and sexual organs setting up violent inflammation. The skin is also markedly affected, a severe vesicular rash developing with intense itching. This is a valuable remedy in nephritis and cystitis typified by frequent attempts at urination, the urine itself containing blood as a rule. It may be indicated in certain postpartum inflammations and burning vesicular eczemas.

Carbo Vegetabilis. Vegetable Charcoal.
Potencies are prepared by trituration and subsequent dilution in alcohol.

Various tissues of the body have a marked affinity with this substance. The circulatory system is particularly affected leading to lack of oxygenation with a corresponding increase of carbon dioxide in the blood and tissues. This is turn leads to a lack of resistance to infections and to haemorrhages of dark blood which does not readily coagulate. Coldness of the body surface supervenes. When potentised this is a very useful remedy in all cases of collapse. Pulmonary congestions will benefit and it restores warmth and strength in cases of circulatory weakness. It acts more on the venous than on the arterial circulation. It could prove useful in some forms of rumenal stasis and bloat resulting from a sluggish portal circulation.

Caulophyllum. Blue Cohosh. N.O. Berberidaceae.
The ⌀ is prepared from trituration of the root dissolved in alcohol.

This plant produces pathological states related to the female genital system. Extraordinary rigidity of the *os uteri* is set up leading to difficulties at parturition. Early abortions may occur due to uterine debility. These may be accompanied by fever and thirst. There is a tendency to retention of afterbirth with possible bleeding from the uterus. In potentised form this remedy will revive labour pains and could be used as an alternative to pituitrin injections once the os is open. It will be found useful in ringwomb and also in cases of uterine twist or displacement. In these cases it should be given frequently for three or four doses, e.g. hourly intervals. In animals which have had previous miscarriages it will help in establishing a normal pregnancy while post-partum it is one of the remedies to be considered for retained afterbirth.

Causticum. Potassium Hydroxide.
This substance is prepared by the distillation of a mixture of equal parts of slaked lime and potassium bisulphate.

The main affinity is with the neuro-muscular system producing weakness and paresis of both types of muscle. Symptoms are aggravated by going from a cold atmosphere to a warm one. It may be of use in bronchitic conditions of older animals and in those which develop small sessile warts. It appears to have an antidotal effect in cases of lead poisoning and could be used in this connection as an adjunct to versenate injections.

Chelidonium. Greater Celandine. N.O. Papaveraceae.
The ⊘ is prepared from the whole plant, fresh at the time of flowering.

A specific action on the liver is produced by this plant. There is general lethargy and indisposition. The tongue is usually coated a dirty yellow and signs of jaundice may be seen in other visible mucous membranes. The liver is constantly upset with the production of clay-coloured stools. Because of its marked hepatic action it should be remembered when dealing with disturbances associated with a sluggish liver action. It may be of use in photosensitisation if signs of jaundice occur.

Cinchona Officinalis. China Officinalis. Peruvian Bark.
N.O. Rubiaceae.
The ⊘ is prepared from the dried bark dissoved in alcohol.

This plant is commonly referred to as 'China' and is the source of quinine. Large doses tend to produce toxic changes, e.g. nervous sensitivity, impaired leucocyte formation, haemorrhages, fever and diarrhoea. Weakness ensues from loss of body fluids. This remedy should be considered when an animal is suffering from debility or exhaustion after fluid loss, e.g. severe diarrhoea or haemorrhage. It is a useful supportive remedy for this reason in white scour in calves. It is seldom indicated in the earlier stages of acute disease.

Cicuta Virosa. Water Hemlock. N.O. Umbelliferae.
The ⊘ is prepared from the fresh root at the time of flowering.

The central nervous system is principally affected by this plant, spasmodic affections occuring. A characteristic feature is the head and neck twisted to one side accompanied by violence of one kind or another. Aggravation occurs from jarring or sudden movement. The general balance becomes upset and there is a tendency to fall to one side while the head and spine bend backwards. Various conditions of the brain and spinal cord may benefit from this remedy, e.g. cerebro-cortical necrosis, louping-ill and milk fever showing the typical lateral deviation of neck.

Cineraria Maritima. Dusty Miller. N.O. Compositae.
The ∅ is prepared from the whole fresh plant.

The active principle is used mainly as an external application in eye conditions and may have a place in the treatment of New Forest disease. The ∅ should be diluted 1/10.

Cobaltum. The Metal. Cobaltum Chloridum. The Salt.
Both these remedies are used mainly in the 30c potency in the treatment of cobalt deficiency in calves and cows and give good results over a period of a few weeks. The chloride has also been used successfully in the treatment of acetonaemia in cows grazing marginal land or on cobalt deficient pasture.

Colchicum Autumnale. Meadow Saffron. N.O. Liliaceae.
The ∅ is prepared from the bulb.

This plant affects muscular tissues, periosteum and synovial membranes of joints. It possesses also an anti-allergic and anti-inflammatory action which interferes with the natural recuperative powers of the body. Illnesses which may require this remedy are uually acute and severe, accompanied frequently by effusions in the small joints. It has a particular value in the treatment of rumenal bloat when it may have to be repeated at frequent intervals. Autumnal diarrhoea and dysentery also may be helped, the latter accompanied by tympany and tenesmus. One of its guiding symptoms is aversion to food, while complaints requiring it are generally worse from movement.

Colocynthis. Bitter Cucumber. N.O. Cucurbitaceae.
The ∅ is prepared from the fruit and contains a glucoside – colocynthin.

This plant is purgative and causes violent inflammatory lesions of the gastro-intestinal tract. Both onset of and relief from symptoms are abrupt. Diarrhoea is yellowish and forcibly expelled. Relief is obtained by movement while aggravation occurs after eating or drinking. This remedy may be needed in scour of calves associated with the characteristic symptom of arching the back and drawing the hind-legs forward under the abdomen.

Conium Maculatum. Hemlock. N.O. Umbelliferae.
The ∅ is prepared from the fresh plant.

The alkaloid of this plant produces a paralytic action on nerve ganglia, especially the motor nerve endings. This leads to stiffness and a paralysis which tends to travel forward or upward. This remedy is of importance in treating paraplegic conditions and any weakness of hind limbs. Thus it could be indicated in those cases of Milk Fever which have not responded satisfactorily to calcium injection.

Convallaria Majalis. Lily of the Valley. N.O. Liliaceae.
The ∅ is prepared from the fresh plant.

The active principle has the power to increase the quality of the heart's action and this determines its main use as a remedy in congestive heart conditions. It has little action on the heart muscle and is used mainly in valvular disease.

Copaiva. Balsam of Peru. N.O. Leguminosae.
The ∅ is prepared from the balsam.

This substance produces a marked action on mucous membranes, especially those of the urinary and respiratory tracts causing a catarrhal inflammation. This action makes the remedy useful in the treatment of urethritis and cystitis. Pyelonephritis is one of the commoner conditions which could be helped.

Crataegus. Hawthorn. N.O. Rosaceae.
The ∅ is prepared from the ripe fruit.

The active principle produces a fall in blood pressure and brings on dyspnoea. It acts on the heart muscle causing an increase in the number and quality of contractions. The specific action on the heart muscle makes this a particularly useful remedy in the treatment of arrythmic heart conditions.

Crotalus Horridus. Rattlesnake.
The ∅ is prepared from trituration of the venom with lactose and subsequent dilution in glycerine.

This venom produces sepsis, haemorrhages and jaundice with decomposition of blood. The marked action of this poison on the vascular system makes it a valuable remedy in the treatment of many low-grade septic states with circulatory involvement, e.g. puerperal fever and wound infections. Septic conditions are accompanied by oozing of blood from any body orifice and are usually attended by jaundice. It should help in conditions such as adder-bite and clover poisoning.

Croton Tiglium. Croton Oil Seeds. N.O. Euphorbiaceae.
The ⌀ is prepared from the oil obtained from the seeds.

This oil produces violent diarrhoea and skin eruptions causing inflammation with a tendency to vesicle formation. This is one of the many useful remedies for controlling diarrhoea. This is usually accompanied by great urging, the stool being watery. Some forms of calf scour may benefit when other symptoms agree, e.g. a gurgling sound may be heard in the intestines and the urine may be orange-coloured.

Cubeba Officinalis. Cubebs. N.O. Piperaceae.
The ⌀ is prepared from the dried unripe fruit.

The active principle acts on mucous membranes producing a catarrhal inflammation. Those of the uro-genital tract are particularly affected, the urine becoming cloudy and albuminous. It could be of use in urethritis, especially of the bull attended by inflammation of the sheath and swollen testicles, producing a muco-purulent discharge.

Cuprum Aceticum. Copper Acetate.
Potencies are prepared from a solution in distilled water.

This salt produces cramping of muscles, spasms and paralytic conditions. It is used chiefly in the treatment of copper deficiency in calves, especially when accompanied by muscle cramping or stiffness. The arsenate of copper and the metal itself are similarly used. The acetate has also been used succesfully in the treatment of cow pox as a supportive remedy.

Curare. Woorara. Arrow Poison.
The ⌀ is prepared from dilutions in alcohol.

This poison produces muscular paralysis without impairing sensation or consciousness. Reflex action is diminished and a state of motor paralysis sets in. It decreases the output of adrenaline and brings about a state of nervous debility. It could have a part to play in the treatment of some forms of recumbency in the cow where consciousness is retained, e.g. in the 'Downer Cow' syndrome as a supportive remedy. Muscular dystrophy in calves could also benefit.

Digitalis Purpurea. Foxglove. N.O. Scrophulariaceae.
The ∅ is prepared from the leaves.

The active principle of the foxglove causes marked slowness of the heart's action, the pulse being weak and irregular. This is a commonly used remedy in heart conditions helping to regulate the beat and producing a stable pulse. By increasing the output of the heart when used in low potencies it aids valvular function. This in turn increases the output of urine and helps reduce oedema. It could, therefore, be of value in treating conditions such as Fog Fever which is usually attended by an increase in bronchial mucus.

Drosera Rotundifolia. Sundew. N.O. Droseraceae.
The ∅ is prepared from the fresh plant.

The lymphatic and pleural systems together with synovial membranes are all affected by this plant. The laryngeal area is also subject to inflammatory processes, any stimulus producing a hypersensitive reaction. In cattle practice its use is restricted to pulmonary and laryngeal conditions, principally pleurisy with dry cough, some forms of pneumonia and upper tracheitis. It has given good results in virus pneumonia in calves, one outbreak in the author's experience responding alone to this remedy.

Dulcamara. Woody Nightshade. N.O. Solanaceae.
The ∅ is prepared from the green stems and leaves before flowering.

This plant belongs to the same family as Belladonna, Hyoscyamus and Stramonium. Tissue affinities are with mucous membranes, glands and kidneys, producing inflammatory changes and interstitial haemorrhages. This remedy may benefit those conditions which arise as a result of exposure to wet and cold, especially when damp evenings follow a warm day. Such conditions commonly occur in autumn and diarrhoea occuring then may benefit. It has proved useful in the treatment of ringworm and could have a beneficial action on large fleshy warts.

Echinacea Angustifolia. Rudbeckia. N.O. Compositae.
The ⌀ is prepared from the whole plant.

Acute toxaemias with septic involvement of various tissues come within the sphere of action of this plant. It is a valuable remedy in the treatment of post-partum puerperal conditions where sepsis is evident. Generalised septic states having their origin in infected bites or stings will also benefit. This remedy acts best in low decimal potencies.

Euphrasia Officinalis. Eyebright. N.O. Scrophulariaceae.
The ⌀ is prepared from the whole plant.

The active principle acts mainly on the conjunctival mucous membrane producing lachrymation. The cornea is also affected, opacities being common. This is one of the most useful remedies in the treatment of a variety of eye conditions, principally conjunctivitis and corneal ulcerations. Internal treatment should be supplemented by its use externally as a lotion diluted 1/10. It should prove useful in New Forest disease.

Ferrum Iodatum. Iodide of Iron.
Potencies are prepared from trituration of crystals subsequently dissolved in alcohol.

This salt is chiefly of interest as a remedy for iron deficiency associated with respiratory distress, mucous discharges containing blood being present. Metallic iron (Ferrum Metallicum) and chloride of iron (Ferrum Muriaticum) are also used in the treatment of iron deficiency, the former particulaly for calves and younger animals and the latter more indicated when heart symptoms such as weak thready pulse are present.

Ferrum Phosphoricum. Ferric Phosphate.
Potencies are prepared from a solution in distilled water.

Febrile conditions in general are associated with this salt. It is frequently used in the early stages of inflammatory conditions which develop less rapidly than those calling for Aconitum. Throat involvement is often the key to its selection. Pulmonary congestions may call for its use if haemorrhages are also present.

Ficus Religiosa. Pakur. N.O. Moraceae.
The ∅ is prepared from fresh leaves in alcohol.

Haemorrhages of various kinds are associated with the toxic effects of this plant. Any condition which produces bleeding of a bright red character may indicate the need for this remedy. It could be of value in Coccidiosis, but generally respiratory rather than digestive upsets determine its use. It may prove of value in Bracken Poisoning.

Fluoricum Acidum. Hydrofluoric Acid.
Potencies are prepared by distilling calcium fluoride with sulphuric acid.

It has an action on most tissues producing deep-seated ulcers and lesions of a destructive nature. It has been used successfully in the treatment of Actinomycosis and in ulcerative conditions of the mouth and throat. Any necrotic condition of bone is likely to benefit.

Gelsemium Sempervirens. Yellow Jasmine. N.O. Loganiaceae.
The ∅ is prepared from the bark of the root.

The affinity of this plant is with the nervous system producing varying degrees of motor paralysis. This remedy has proved helpful as a supportive measure in Hypomagnesaemia, aiding restoration of normal movement. Single paralysis of different nerves, e.g. the radial may also benefit. Conditions which call for its use are usually attended by weakness and muscle tremors.

Glonoinum. Nitro-Glycerine.
Potencies are prepared from dilutions in alcohol.

This substance has an affinity with the brain and circulatory system causing sudden and violent convulsions and also congestions in the arterial system leading to throbbing and pulsations, seen in superficial vessels. It will be found of use in brain conditions arising from over-exposure to heat or the effects of the sun. It may also help the convulsions associated with Hypomagnesaemia and allied conditions.

Graphites. Black Lead.
Potencies are prepared from triturations dissolved in alcohol.

This form of carbon has an affinity with skin and hooves. Eruptions are common and its action on connective tissue tends to produce fibrotic conditions associated with malnutrition. Loss of hair occurs while purply moist eruptions ooze a sticky discharge. Abrasions develop into ulcers which may suppurate. Favourable sites for eczema are in the bends of joints and behind the ears.

Hamamelis Virginica. Witch Hazel. N.O. Hamamelidaceae.
The ⌀ is prepared from fresh bark of twigs and roots.

This plant has an affinity with the venous circulation producing congestions and haemorrhages. The action on the veins is one of relaxation with consequent engorgement. Any condition showing venous engorgement or congestion with passive haemorrhage should show improvement from the use of this remedy.

Hecla Lava. Hecla.
Potencies are prepared from trituration of the volcanic ash. Present in this ash are the substances which accompany lava formation, viz. Alumina, Lime and Silica.

Lymphoid tissue and the skeleton are areas which show the greatest affinity for this substance. The remedy is useful in the treatment of exostoses or tumours of the facial bones and in caries arising from dental disease. It has proved successful in the treatment of actinomycosis affecting the maxillary and mandibular bones. It should help in the treatment of bony tumours generally.

Hepar Sulphuris Calcareum. Impure Calcium Sulphide.
This substance is prepared by burning crude calcium carbonate with flowers of sulphur. Potencies are then prepared from the triturated ash.

This remedy is associated with suppurative processes producing conditions which are extemely sensitive to touch. It causes catarrhal and purulent inflammation of the mucous membranes of the respiratory and alimentary tracts with involvement of the skin and lymphatic system. This remedy has a wide range of action and should be considered in any suppurative process showing extreme sensitivity to touch indicating acute pain, e.g. acute summer mastitis. Low potencies of this remedy promote suppuration while high potencies – 200c and upwards may abort the purulent process and promote resolution.

Hydrastis Canadensis. Golden Seal. N.O. Ranunculaceae.
The ⌀ is prepared from the fresh root.

Mucous membranes are affected by this plant, a catarrhal inflammation being established. Secretions generally are thick and yellow. Any catarrhal condition resulting in a muco-purulent discharge will come within the scope of this remedy, e.g. mild forms of metritis or sinusitis.

Hydrocotyle Asiatica. Indian Pennywort. N.O. Umbelliferae.
The ⌀ is prepared from the whole plant.

The main affinity of this plant is with the skin and female genital system. It also has a lesser effect on the action of the liver. Skin conditions showing thickening of epidermis and roughening come within its sphere of action.

Hyoscyamus Niger. Henbane. N.O. Solanaceae.
The ⌀ is prepared from the fresh plant.

The active principle disturbs the central nervous system producing symptoms of brain excitement and mania. This remedy has proved effective in the treatment of Grass Tetany preventing brain damage supervening. Conditions which call for its use are not accompanied by inflammation (cf. Belladonna).

Hypericum Perforatum. St. John's Wort. N.O. Hyperiaceae.
The ⌀ is prepared from the whole fresh plant.

The active principle is capable of causing sensitivity to light on some skins in the absence of melanin pigment. The main affinity is with the nervous system causing hypersensitivity. Sloughing and necrosis of skin may take place. This remedy is of prime importance in the treatment of lacerated wounds where nerve endings are damaged. In spinal injuries, especially of the coccygeal area, it gives good results. The specific action on nerves suggests its use in tetanus where, given early after injury, it helps prevent the spread of toxin. It can be used externally for lacerated wounds along with Calendula, both in a strength of 1/10. It has been found useful in the treatment of photosensitisation and similar allergies.

Iodium. Iodine. The Element.
Potencies are prepared from the tincture prepared by dissolving the element in alcohol. A 1% tincture is the strength used in preparation.

In large doses – Iodism – sinuses and eyes are at first involved leading to conjunctivitis and bronchitis. Iodine has a special affinity with the thyroid gland. Weakness and atrophy of muscles may follow excessive intake. The skin becomes dry and withered looking and the appetite becomes voracious. Conditions which show a characteristic oppositeness of symptoms, e.g. tissue hyperplasia or atrophy may need this remedy. It may be of use in ovarian dysfunction when the ovaries appear small and shrunken on rectal examination. It is a useful gland remedy and its specific relation to the thyroid should not be forgotten.

Ipecacuanha. N.O. Rubiaceae.
The ∅ is prepared from the dried root. Emetine, an alkaloid is its principal constituent.

This plant is associated with haemorrhages and has found a use in the treatment of post-partum bleeding where the blood comes in gushes. Blood in the milk after calving will generally yield to this remedy. Emetine has a purgative action and the remedy is one of the chief among those used in the treatment of Coccidiosis in calves. Some forms of white scour may also benefit, particularly those showing tenesmus with greenish stools.

Kali Arsenicum. Fowler's Solution. Potassium Arsenite.
Dilutions of this salt provide the ∅·

The main action which concerns us in cattle practice is exerted on the skin, a dry scaly eczema with itching being established. Slow-healing ulcers appear with fissures in the region of the elbows and hocks. It is a good general skin remedy.

Kali Bichromicum. Potassium Dichromate.
Potencies are prepared from a solution in distilled water.

This salt acts on the mucous membranes of the stomach, intestines and respiratory tract with lesser involvement of other organs. Feverish states are absent. The action on the mucous membranes produces a catarrhal discharge of a tough stringy character with a yellow colour. This particular type of discharge is a strong guiding symptom for its use. It could be used in Broncho-Pneumonia, Sinusitis and Pyelonephritis. It has been used successfully in Cow Pox where lesions take the form of round shallow ulcers with smooth edges and a pronounced yellow centre.

Kali Carbonicum. Potassium Carbonate.
Potencies are prepared from a solution in distilled water.

This salt is found in all plants and in the soil, the colloid material of cells containing potassium.

It produces a generalised weakness which is common to other potassium salts. Feverish states are absent. It could be a useful convalescent remedy.

Kali Chloricum. Potassium Chlorate.
Potencies are prepared from a solution in distilled water.

The urinary organs are chiefly affected, producing a blood-stained and albuminous urine with a high phosphate content.

Kali Hydriodicum. Potassium Iodide.
Potencies are prepared from triturations dissolved in alcohol.

This important drug produces an acrid watery discharge from the eyes and also acts on fibrous and connective tissue. Glandular swellings also appear. This is a widely used remedy in various conditions showing the typical eye and respiratory symptoms, e.g. in the early stages of New Forest disease it has proved most beneficial in preventing extension of the process. It is one of the main remedies to be considered in the treatment of Actinobacillosis (Wooden Tongue), especially with involvement of the sub-maxillary glands.

Lachesis. Bushmaster. Surucucu Snake.
Trituration of venom dissolved in alcohol is the source of the solution which yields the potencies.

This venom produces decomposition of blood rendering it more fluid. There is a strong tendency to haemorrhage and sepsis with profound prostration. This is a useful remedy for Adder bites helping to prevent septic complications and reducing swelling. It is particularly valuable if the throat develops inflammation causing left-sided swelling which may involve the parotid gland. Where haemorrhage takes place the blood is dark and does not clot readily while the skin surrounding any lesion assumes a purplish appearance. Mastitis showing bluish or purplish discolouration of skin, especially on the left quarters, should improve under this remedy.

Lathyrus Sativus. Chick Pea. N.O. Leguminosae.
The ⊘ is prepared from the flower and the pods.

This plant affects the anterior columns of the spinal cord producing paralysis of the lower extremities. Nerve power generally is weakened. It should be considered in recumbent conditions associated with mineral deficiencies and in any state involving nerve weakness leading to local paralysis.

Ledum Palustre. Marsh Tea. Wild Rosemary. N.O. Ericaceae.
The ⌀ is prepared from the whole plant.

The active principle produces tetanus-like symptoms with twitching of muscles. It is one of the main remedies for punctured wounds, especially when the surrounding area becomes cold and discoloured. Insect bites respond well. Also injuries to the eye.

Lobelia Inflata. Indian Tobacco. N.O. Lobeliaceae.
The ⌀ is prepared from the dried leaves with subsequent dilution in alcohol.

The active principle acts as a vaso-motor stimulant impeding respiration and producing symptoms of inappetance and relaxation of muscles. It is of value in emphysematous conditions and as a general convalescent remedy.

Lycopodium Clavatum. Club Moss. N.O. Lycopodiaceae.
The ⌀ is prepared from trituration of the spores and dilution in alcohol. The spores are inactive until triturated and potentised.

The active principle acts chiefly on the digestive and renal systems. The respiratory system is also affected, pneumonia being a frequent complication. There is general lack of gastric function and very little food will satisfy. The abdomen becomes bloated with tenderness over the liver. The glycogenic function of the liver is interfered with. This is a very useful remedy in various digestive, urinary and respiratory conditions, a guiding symptom being that complaints frequently show an aggravation in the late afternoon or early evening. It is the first remedy of choice in the digestive form of acetonaemia while its action on the skin suggests its use in alopecia.

Magnesia Phosphorica. Phosphate of Magnesium.
Potencies are prepared from trituration of the salt in solution.

This salt acts on muscles producing a cramping effect with spasm. It is a valuable remedy to be remembered as supportive treatment in hypomagnesaemia where its prompt use will limit the tendency to brain damage and help fix the element in the system, as otherwise it may be quickly excreted.

Melilotus. Sweet Clover. N.O. Leguminosae.
The ⊘ is prepared from the whole fresh plant.

This plant is associated with profuse haemorrhages. Clover contains a haemolytic agent which prevents clotting of blood after mechanical injuries. This is more likely to happen if animals are fed mouldy hay. It should be remembered as a possibly useful remedy in conditions like bracken poisoning and in haematomas and subcutaneous bleeding of unknown origin.

Mercurius. Mercurius Solubilis. Mercury.
Potencies are prepared from triturations and dilutions in alcohol.

This metal affects most organs and tissues producing cellular degeneration with consequent anaemia. Salivation accompanies most complaints and gums become spongy and bleed easily. Diarrhoea is common, stools being slimy and blood-stained. Conditions calling for its use are worse in the period sunset to sunrise.

Mercurius Corrosivus. Mercuric Chloride. Corrosive Sublimate.
Potencies are prepared from triturations and subsequent dilution.

This salt has a somewhat similar action to mercurius sol., but generally the symptoms produced are more severe. It produces severe tenesmus of the lower bowel leading to dysentery and also has a destructive action on kidney tissue. Discharges from mucous surfaces assume a greenish tinge. It could be of value in severe cases of Coccidiosis.

Mercurius Cyanatus. Cyanate of Mercury.
Potencies are prepared from triturations and dilutions.

This particular salt produces an action similar to that associated with bacterial toxins. A haemorrhagic tendency with prostration is a common feature. Ulceration of the mucous membranes of the mouth and throat commonly occur which suggests its use in calf diphtheria. A greyish membrane surrounds these ulcerated surfaces. The pharyngeal area is one of the main regions to be affected, redness of the membrane preceding necrosis in the later stages.

Mercurius Dulcis. Calomel. Mercurous Chloride.
Potencies are prepared from triturations and dilution.

This salt has an affinity with the ear and liver especially. Hepatitis with jaundice may result. It is worth considering as a possibly useful remedy in mild forms of cirrhosis.

Mercurius Iodatus Flavus. Yellow Iodide of Mercury.
Potencies are prepared from triturations in dilution.

Mercurous Iodide produces a tendency to glandular induration with attendant coating of the tongue. Sub-maxillary and parotid glands become swollen, more pronounced on the right side. Various swellings of glandular tissue come within the sphere of this remedy, e.g. parotitis and lymphadenitis generally. It could be of value in actinobacillosis when lesions attack on the right side.

Mercurius Iodatus Ruber. Red Iodide of Mercury.
Potencies are prepared from triturations of the salt.

Mercuric Iodide also has a tendency to produce glandular swellings, but in this case the left side of the throat is involved. Stiffness of neck muscles may be a prominent symptom.

Millefolium. Yarrow. N.O. Compositae.
The ⊘ is prepared from the whole plant.

Haemorrhages occur from various parts from the action of this plant. The blood is bright red. It could be of use in acute mastitis showing blood in the milk and tenderness of teats. It should also increase the amount of milk.

Murex Purpurea. Purple Fish.
The ⊘ is prepared from the dried secretion of the purple gland of one of the Murex species.

It exerts its action mainly on the female genital system producing irregularities of the oestrus cycle. It has been employed both in anoestrus and for stimulating ovulation, but probably it will give best results in cystic ovary leading to nymphomania.

Muriatic Acid. Hydrochloric Acid.
Potencies are prepared from dilutions, in distilled water.

This acid produces a blood condition analagous to that associated with septic feverish states of a chronic nature. There is a tendency for ulcers to form. The throat becomes dark red and oedematous while ulceration of lips accompanies swollen gums and neck glands.

Natrum Muriaticum. Common Salt. Sodium Chloride.
Potencies are prepared from triturations dissolved in distilled water.

Excessive intake of common salt leads to anaemia, evidenced by dropsy or oedema of various parts. White blood cells are increased while mucous membranes are rendered dry. This is a remedy which is of value in unthrifty conditions arising as a result of anaemia or chronic nephritis. Its use in cattle practice is limited.

Naja Tripudians. Cobra.

Potencies are prepared from trituration of the venom and subsequent dilution in alcohol. Alternatively the ∅ may be prepared by dilution of the pure venom.

This poison produces a bulbar paralysis. Haemorrhages are scanty but oedema is marked. The underlying tissues appear dark purple after a bite, blood-stained fluid being present in large quantities. Loss of limb control supervenes. The heart is markedly affected. It could be of use in angio-neurotic oedema.

Nitricum Acidum. Nitric Acid.

Potencies are prepared from a solution in distilled water.

This acid affects particularly body outlets where skin and mucous membranes meet. It produces ulceration and blisters in the mouth and causes offensive discharges. The ulceration may also affect mucous membranes elsewhere and it has been of benefit in some forms of mucosal disease in calves.

Nux Vomica. Poison Nut. N.O. Loganiaceae.

The ∅ is prepared from the seeds.

Digestive disturbances and congestions are associated with this plant, flatulence and indigestion being commonly encountered. Stools are generally hard. Digestive upsets as a result of too much green food should respond to it and it is a useful remedy to give as a preliminary treatment in cases of plant poisoning. Rumenal stasis is likely to benefit.

Opium. Poppy. N.O. Papaveraceae.

The ∅ is prepared from the powder after trituration.

Opium produces an insensibility of the nervous system with stupor and torpor. There is lack of vital reaction. All complaints are characterised by soporific states. Pupils are contracted and the eyes assume a staring look. This remedy has a limited use in cattle practice and is chiefly used in severe cases of bowel inactivity associated with the characteristic sleepy state.

Palladium. The Metal.
Potencies are prepared from triturations and subsequent dilution in alcohol.

This element produces its main action on the female genital system, especially the ovaries causing an inflammation with a tendency to pelvic peritonitis. The right ovary is more usually affected. It is, therefore, likely to benefit those cows and heifers showing irregular oestrus when dependent on ovarian dysfunction. Pelvic disorders arising as a result of ovaritis should also benefit.

Phosphoricum Acidum. Phosphoric Acid.
Potencies are prepared from a dilution of the acid in distilled water.

This acid produces a debilitating state in which flatulence and diarrhoea are common features. It is of value in helping the metabolism of the young growing animal, especially the dairy calf.

Pulsatilla. Anemone. N.O. Ranunculaceae.
The ∅ is prepared from the entire plant when in flower.

Mucous membranes come within the sphere of action of this plant, thick muco-purulent discharges being produced. It has proved useful in the treatment of ovarian hypofunction and in retained placenta.

Ranunculus Bulbosus. Buttercup. N.O. Ranunculaceae.
The ∅ is prepared from the whole plant.

The action in mainly on muscular tissue and skin producing a hypersensitivity to touch. Skin lesions take the form of papular and vesicular eruptions which may cluster together into over-shaped groups. The remedy could be of value in some forms of Cow pox and allied skin complaints.

Rhododendron. Snow Rose. N.O. Ericaceae.
The ∅ is prepared from the fresh leaves.

This shrub is associated with muscular and joint stiffness. Orchitis is not uncommon with the testicles becoming hard and indurated. It may be of value in such conditions in the bull with accompanying epididymetis.

Rhus Toxicodendron. Poison Oak. N.O. Anacardiaceae.
The ∅ is prepared from the fresh leaves.

The active principles of this tree affect skin and muscles together with mucous membranes and fibrous tissues producing tearing pains and blistery eruptions. Symptoms of stiffness are relieved by movement. Involvement of the skin leads to a reddish rash with vesicles and produces a cellulitis of neighbouring tissues. It could be a useful remedy in muscle and joint conditions which show a characteristic improvement on exercise.

Ruta Graveolens. Rue. N.O. Rutaceae.
The ∅ is prepared from the whole fresh plant.

Ruta produces its action on the periosteum and cartilages with a secondary effect on eyes and uterus. Deposits form around the carpal joints, particularly. It has also a selective action on the lower bowel and rectum and could prove useful in mild forms of rectal prolapse. It has been known to facilitate labour by increasing the tone of uterine contractions.

Sabina. Savine. N.O. Coniferae.
The ∅ is prepared from the oil dissolved in alcohol.

The uterus is the main seat of action producing a tendency to abortion. There is also an action of fibrous tissues and serous membranes. It is associated with haemorrhages of bright red blood which remains fluid. This remedy has its main use in uterine conditions including retained placenta. Persistent post-partum bleeding may also be arrested.

Sanguinaria. Blood Root. N.O. Papaveraceae.
The ∅ is prepared from the fresh root.

An alkaloid – sanguinarine – contained in this plant has an affinity with the circulatory system leading to congestion and redness of skin. The female genital system is affected, inflammation of ovaries occurring. Small cutaneous haemorrhages arise in various sites. Stiffness of fore-legs, especially the left shoulder region may be seen.

Secale Cornutum. Ergot of Rye. N.O. Fungi.
The ∅ is prepared from the fresh fungus.

Ergot produces marked contraction of smooth muscle causing a diminuation of blood supply to various areas. This is particularly seen in peripheral blood vessels, especially of the feet. Stools are dark green alternating with dysentery. Bleeding of dark blood occurs from the uterus with putrid discharges. The skin becomes dry and shrivelled-looking with a tendency for gangrene to form. Because of its circulatory action and its effect on smooth muscle it is useful in some uterine conditions, e.g. post-partum bleeding of dark blood and in any condition with impairment of peripheral circulation.

Sepia Officinalis. Cuttlefish.
Potencies are prepared from trituration of the dried liquid from the ink bag.

Portal congestion and stasis are associated with this substance along with disturbances of function in the female genital system. Prolapse of uterus may occur or a tendency thereto. It will regulate the entire oestrus cycle and should always be given as a routine preliminary remedy in treatment. It has also an action on the skin and has given good results in the treatment of ringworm. Post-partum discharges of various sorts will usually respond. It is also capable of encouraging the natural maternal instinct in those animals which are indifferent or hostile to their offspring.

Silicea. Pure Flint.
Potencies are prepared from triturations dissolved in alcohol.

The main action of this substance is on bone where it is capable of causing caries and necrosis. It also causes abscesses and fistulae of connective tissue with secondary fibrous growths. There is a tendency for all wounds to suppurate. This is a widely used remedy indicated in many suppurative processess of a chronic nature. It gives good results in summer mastitis and will hasten resolution of the udder, by its ability to absorb scar tissue.

Spongia Tosta. Roasted Sponge.
Potencies are prepared from dilutions in alcohol.

This substance produces symptoms related to the respiratory and cardiac spheres. The lymphatic system is also affected. The thyroid gland becomes enlarged. The general action on glands suggest its use in Lymphadenitis. It is principally used as a heart remedy after respiratory infections.

Stramonium. Thorn Apple. N.O. Solanaceae.
The ⊘ is prepared from the fresh plant in flower.

The active principle of this shrub produces its main action on the central nervous system giving a staggering gait dependent on brain involvement. There is a tendency to fall forward. Pupils of the eye become dilated with a fixed staring look. There are also convulsive movements of the fore-limbs and isolated groups of muscles. This remedy has a role to play in helping to control the brain symptoms of conditions such as hypomagnesaemia. Other conditions which may benefit are cerebro-cortical necrosis and the nervous form of acetonaemia.

Strophanthus. Onage. N.O. Apocynaceae.
The ∅ is prepared from the seeds dissolved in alcohol.

This shrub produces an increase in the contractile power of striped muscle. It acts especially on the heart increasing systole. The amount of urine passed is increased and albuminuria may be present. This is a useful heart remedy to help remove oedema. It is a safe and useful diuretic especially for the older animal.

Strychninum. Strychnine. Alkaloid Contained in Nux Vomica.
Potencies are prepared from solutions in distilled water

This alkaloid stimulates the motor centres of the spinal cord and increases the depth of respirations. All reflexes are rendered more active and pupils become dilated. Rigidity of muscles occurs especially of the neck and back with jerking and twitching of limbs. Muscle tremors and tetanic convulsions set in rapidly. This remedy may prove useful in severe forms of hypomagnesaemia or cerebro-cortical necrosis if the specific symptoms are present.

Sulphur. The Element.
Potencies are prepared from trituration and subsequent dilution in alcohol.

This element has a wide range of action, but in cattle practice it is chiefly used in skin conditions such as mange and eczema and also as an inter-current remedy to aid the action of other remedies.

Symphytum. Comfrey. N.O. Boraginaceae.
The ∅ is prepared from the fresh plant.

The root of this plant produces a substance which stimulates growth of epithelium on ulcerated surfaces and hastens union of bone in fractures. It should always be given as a routine remedy in fractures as an aid to healing. This will not often be indicated in cattle practice, but it could be helpful in the treatment of a valuable animal. Together with other vulneraries like arnica it is indicated in the treatment of injuries in general. It is also a prominent eye remedy.

Tellurium. The Metal.
Potencies are prepared from triturations dissolved in alcohol.

This element exerts an influence on skin, eyes and ears. A pustular conjunctivitis may arise and the skin of the outer ear may show eczematous eruptions. Skin lesions tend to assume a ring-like shape and to appear symmetrically on both sides of the body. Because of this action it has been used successfully in the treatment of ringworm.

Terebinthinae. Oil of Turpentine.
Potencies are prepared from a solution in alcohol.

Haemorrhages are produced from various surfaces, urinary symptoms predominating. There is difficulty in urinating and blood commonly occurs in the urine. Bleeding may also take place in the uterus, especially after parturition. It is principally used in acute nephritis associated with haematuria and a sweet-smelling urine. This odour has been likened to that of violets. It also has a use in the treatment of gaseous bloat when low potencies will help.

Thlaspi Bursa Pastoralis. Shepherd's Purse. N.O. Cruciferae.
The ⊘ is prepared from the fresh plant.

This plant produces haemorrhages with a uric acid diathesis. It favours expulsion of blood clots from the uterus and is indicated after miscarriage. There is frequency of urination, the urine being heavy and turbid with a reddish sediment. Cystitis is commonly seen with blood-stained urine.

Thuja Occidentalis. Arbor Vitae. N.O. Coniferae.
The ⊘ is prepared from fresh twigs.

Thuja produces a condition which favours the formation of warty growths and tumours. It acts mainly on the skin and uro-genital system. Warts and herpetic eruptions develop, the neck and abdomen being the favourite sites. This remedy is of great importance in the treatment of skin conditions accompanied by the development of warty growths which bleed easily. Papillomatous warts are especially influenced and this action may be enhanced by the external application of the remedy in ⌀ form.

Thyroidium. Thyroid Gland.
Potencies are prepared from triturations and dilution in alcohol.

Anaemia, emaciation and muscular weakness are associated with excess of thyroid secretion. There is dilation of pupils with prominence. Heart rate is increased. This remedy may be of use in the treatment of alopecia and allied skin conditions.

Trinitrotoluene.
Potencies are prepared from a solution in distilled water.

This substance exerts a destructive influence on red blood cells causing haemolysis with consequent loss of haemoglobin. This produces anaemia and this is the principle of treatment by this remedy. It could be of use in babesiasis and similar conditions.

Urtica Urens. Stinging Nettle. N.O. Urticaceae.
The ⌀ is prepared from the fresh plant.

The nettle causes agalactia with a tendency to the formation of calculi. There is a general uric acid diathesis with urticarial swellings being present on the skin. There is diminished secretion of urine. The mammary glands become enlarged with surrounding oedema. This is a very useful remedy in various renal and skin conditions. In the treatment of uric acid tendencies it acts by thickening the urine which contains increased deposits of urates. It helps promote normal urination and will increase the flow of milk after parturition.

Uva Ursi. Bearberry. N.O. Ericaceae.
The ⌀ is prepared from dried leaves and fruit.

The active principles are associated with disturbances of the urinary system. Cystitis commonly occurs and the urine may contain blood, pus and mucus. Kidney involvement is usually confined to the pelvis causing a purulent inflammation. This is one of the main remedies used in the treatment of cystitis and pyelonephritis.

Veratrum Album. White Hellebore. N.O. Liliaceae.
The ⌀ is prepared from root stocks.

A picture of collapse is presented by the action of this plant.

Extremities become cold and signs of cyanosis appear. Purging occurs, the watery diarrhoea being accompanied by exhaustion. This is a useful remedy in some forms of scour in calves. The body surface quickly becomes cold and the stools are greenish. Signs of abdominal pain precede the onset of diarrhoea, e.g. kicking at abdomen with an accompanying abdominal tympany.

Viburnum Opulis. Water Elder. Cranberry. N.O. Caprifoliaceae.
The ∅ is prepared from the fresh bark.

Muscular cramps are associated with the action of this plant. The female genital system is markedly affected, chiefly the uterus producing a tendency to abortion in the first quarter of pregnancy, sterility being a common sequel. It is principally used in the treatment of animals with a history of repeated miscarriages.

Vipera. Common Viper.
Potencies are prepared from diluted venom.

This poison causes paresis of the hind limbs with a tendency to paralysis. Symptoms extend upwards. Skin and subcutaneous tissues become swollen after a bite with livid tongue and swollen lips developing. Disturbances of liver function produces a jaundice of visible mucous membranes. Inflammation of veins occurs with attendant oedema. Oedematous states arising from venous congestion provide conditions suitable for its use and it should be remembered as a possibly useful remedy in liver dysfunction.

Zincum Metallicum. Zinc. The Metal.
Potencies are prepared from trituration with subsequent dilution in alcohol.

This element produces a state of anaemia with a decrease in the number of red cells. There is a tendency to fall towards the left side with weakness and trembling of muscles. It is a useful remedy in suppressed feverish states accompanied by anaemia and may prove useful in brain conditions showing typical symptoms.

Nosodes and Oral Vaccines.
Reference to nosodes and oral vaccines has already been made in the preface to this book, and it is only necessary to add that all disease products are rendered innocuous after the third centesimal potency which is equivalent to a strength or dilution of 1/1,000,000. They are used in the 30c. potency.

Bacillinum
This remedy is prepared from tuberculous material. It has a limited use in cattle practice, but it is extremely useful in the treatment of ringworm and similar skin diseases.

Carcinosin
The Nosode of Carcinoma.
   This little used remedy in cattle practice can be helpful in cases of glandular enlargements accompanied by feverish states.

Corynebacterium Pyogenes.
This oral vaccine is prepared from the bacterium which is associated with summer mastitis in the dry cow or from diseased material and discharges from the udder. It can be used both prophylactically and therapeutically.

E. Coli Nosode and Oral Vaccine.
Prepared from various strains of E. Coli. It has been found in practice that the strain which has given the most consistent results is the one which was prepared originally from a human source. Both treatment and prevention of coli-bacillosis come within its range and also the specific form of mastitis associated with E. Coli infection.

Folliculinum.
The nosode prepared from the corpus luteum is used chiefly in the treatment of various ovarian and allied conditions.

Oopherinum.
This is the actual ovarian hormone. Ovarian troubles come within its sphere of action, e.g. sterility dependent on ovarian dysfunction. It also has been used in some forms of skin disorder thought to be associated with hormone imbalance.

Psorinum. Scabies Vesicle.
This is a valuable skin remedy. It is not often called for in cattle practice, but should be kept in mind as a possibly useful addition to the more commonly used remedies. Ringworm may respond as well as other conditions attended by dry coat and great itching.

Pyrogenium. Pyrogen.

This nosode is prepared from decaying animal protein. Despite its origin it is an extremely valuable remedy in the treatment of septicaemic or toxaemic states where vital reserves are low. One of the main indications for its use is illness attended by a high temperature alternating with a weak thready pulse, or alternatively a low temperature with a firm pulse. All discharges and septic states are extremely offensive. It could have a vital part to play in puerperal feverish conditions, and has been used in retained afterbirth after abortions.

Salmonella Nosode and Oral Vaccine.

Prepared from the common Salmonella organisms associated with this disease in calves and used both prophylactically and therapeutically.

Streptococcus Nosode and Oral Vaccine.

Prepared from strains of haemolytic streptococci. It is used in various infections associated with these bacteria. Joint-ill in calves has responded well and it also has a prominent part to play in the control of mastitis.

Sycotic Co. One of the Bowel Nosodes.

This is one of a group of nosodes prepared from the non-lactose fermenting bacilli found in the large intestine. Each one is related to certain homoeopathic remedies and used mainly in conjunction with them. They are also used by themselves. Sycotic Co. has been used successfully in intestinal conditions producing catarrhal inflammation on mucous membranes, e.g. in the treatment of coccidiosis in calves.

Tuberculinum Aviare.

Avian sources provide the material for this nosode.

This nosode may prove useful in the treatment of some forms of pneumonia, especially in calves, along with indicated remedies. Chronic conditions are the most likely to benefit.

Index

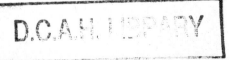

117, 119, 120, 122, 123, 126, 129:
arterial, 1; bright red blood, 36,
126; dark blood, 109; internal, 45;
interstitial, 114; passive, 36, 117;
petechial, 36; scanty, 124;
venous, 1
Hair, loss of, 92–93, 117
Hamamelis Virginica. Witch Hazel,
117
Head: extended, 56; pain in, 54;
restriction of, 96; retraction of,
23, 96; swelling of h. bones, 58;
twisting of, 110, 111
Head pressing, 24, 25
Head shaking and rolling, 3, 20, 23,
24, 25, 33, 42, 70; raising and
lowering of, 40
Heart: increased quality of action,
112; increased rate, 11, 13, 24, 37,
46, 47, 64, 88, 96, 130; murmur,
13; slowness of action, 114;
symptoms, 45; variation in
sounds, 13; very rapid action, 14
Heart muscle: attacks on, 97;
dilation of, 13; increase in
number and quality of
contractions, 112; relieving stress
on, 14; weakness of, 13
Heat: irregular periods, 78;
over-exposure to, 116; silent, 101
Heat exhaustion, 53; symptoms, 54,
treatment, 54
Heat Prostration, 53
Hecla Lava. Hecla, 117
Hepar Sulphuris Calcareum.
Impure Calcium Sulphide, 117
Hepatic disturbance, 9
Hepatitis, 5, 122: Necrotic, 22:
symptoms, 22; treatment, 22
High-stepping, exaggerated, 70
Hind-legs, drawing forward of, 112
Hooves, distortion of, 28
Hydrastis Canadensis. Golden Seal,
118
Hydrocotyle Asiatica. Indian
Pennywort, 118
Hyoscyamus Niger. Henbane, 118
Hyper-excitability, 40, 41, 48
Hypericum Perforatum. St. John's
Wort, 118
Hyperkeratosis, 92: symptoms,
92–3; treatment, 93; chronic,
92–3

Hyperplasia, Interdigital, 29:
symptoms, 29; treatment, 29
Hypersensitivity, 118
Hypertrophy, 2
Hypercalcaemia, 40: Parturient, 41:
symptoms, 41–2; treatment, 42
Hypermagnesaemia, 101, 104, 107,
116, 121, 128

Incoordination, 48, 65, 66, 86, 103;
of gait, 70
Indigestion, 60, 124; Acute, 18:
symptoms, 19; treatment, 19;
simple, 19
Indisposition, 110
Infection, 30: necrotic, 29;
septicaemic, 30
Infectious Bovine Rhinotrachitis,
66: symptoms, 66; treatment,
66–7
Infectious Keratitis, 90: symptoms,
91, treatment, 91; prevention of,
91
Infertility, 72, 108: in cow, 76–80;
main causes of, 77
Inflammation, 33, 34, 118:
conjunctival, 2; of heart, 14; of
intestines, 86, 133; of laryngeal
area, 4; of larynx, 67; of salivary
glands, 18; of vein, 14, 131;
resolution in, 64; suppurative, 3;
vesicular of genital tract, 71
Intestines: gurgling in, 113;
inflammation of, 86, 133; mucous
membranes of, 88
Iodium. Iodine, 118–19
Ipecacuanha, 119
Iron deficiency, 115
Irritation, 29
Itch, *see* Mange
Itching, 18, 33, 34, 119; intense,
109, 132

Jaundice, 15, 17, 22, 33, 45, 46, 47,
55, 92, 105, 110, 113, 122, 131
Jaws: champing of, 24; swellings on,
58
Joint: carpus, 84; deformities in, 88;
degeneration, 26; extension of,
26; fetlock, 84; flexion of, 26;
hock, 84; knee, 88; palpation of,
26; pastern, infection of, 27;
shoulder, 84; stiffness in, 125;